‘Ofra Eshel’s *Reinventing Psychoanalysis for the Great Unknown: The Never-Ending Challenge* is a magnificent tribute to her work in which she reinvents psychoanalysis in a form that is suited to treating severe traumatic states and other forms of psychic difficulty previously unreachable. She delves deeply into *her experience with the patient* to accompany him or her through the depths of darkness in which the patient has lived alone and consequently without the possibility of continuing the journey into becoming oneself. This is an invaluable book that marks the frontier of contemporary psychoanalysis.’

Thomas Ogden, *author of* What Alive Means *and* Coming to Life in the Consulting Room

‘In this remarkable new volume, Ofra Eshel deepens and expands her groundbreaking original ideas on analytic oneness, exploring its vital role in psychoanalytic work at the deepest levels of the mind. With illuminating commentaries by distinguished psychoanalytic thinkers, the book ventures courageously into the unknown frontiers of analytic experience—where challenge, mystery, and transformation intertwine. Eshel’s notion of “quantum interconnectedness” opens a visionary path, suggesting that psychoanalysis, like quantum physics, can transcend the boundaries of conventional science. Her striking clinical illustrations exemplify her rare capacity to think, feel, and write from within the very heart of psychoanalysis.’

João Carlos Braga, *MD, PhD, training and supervising analyst, the Brazilian Psychoanalytic Society of São Paulo, and Brazilian Psychoanalytic Society of Curitiba, Brazil*

AF736327

Reinventing Psychoanalysis for the Great Unknown

This book explores extreme experiences in psychoanalysis and examines how to work with and understand such experiences both theoretically and practically.

It invites readers into new, transformative quantum frontiers of psychoanalytic thought and clinical experience. Taking her profound work as the heart of the conversation, Eshel and a distinguished range of authors examine the essence of the great unknown in diverse realms of psychoanalysis—from massively traumatic states and enigmatic telepathic dreams to the sudden, shattering death of a patient. They focus on the decisive shift from classical psychoanalysis and its epistemological boundaries to the traumatic, the catastrophic, and the unknowable—charting an ontological–experiential, quantum frontier of analytic work. Inspired by Winnicott and Bion, yet reaching beyond them, these contributions open both mind and heart to a dimension of radical presence and deeply transformative forms of analytic oneness, making possible encounters with even the most seemingly unreachable patients.

This is essential reading for psychoanalysts and psychotherapists seeking to extend the reach of psychoanalytic treatment and to work with some of the most difficult clinical situations.

Ofra Eshel is a faculty member and training and supervising analyst of the Israel Psychoanalytic Society and a fellow of the IPA. She is an honorary member of the New Center for Psychoanalysis, Los Angeles. She founded and heads the post-graduate track "Winnicott, Bion, and Independent Psychoanalysis: Radical Breakthrough" at Tel Aviv University, and also (in 2024) the advanced program "Radical Breakthroughs in Contemporary Psychoanalysis" in Beijing, China. Her book, *The Emergence of Analytic Oneness* (Routledge, 2019), has been translated into Chinese, Brazilian Portuguese, and Hebrew, with Spanish and Russian translations in progress.

PSYCHOANALYSIS IN A NEW KEY BOOK SERIES

DONNEL STERN

Series Editor

When music is played in a new key, the melody does not change, but the notes that make up the composition do change in the context of continuity, continuity that perseveres through change. Psychoanalysis in a New Key publishes books that share the aims psychoanalysts have always had, but that approach them differently. The books in the series are not expected to advance any particular theoretical agenda, although to this date most have been written by analysts from the Interpersonal and Relational orientations.

The most important contribution of a psychoanalytic book is the communication of something that nudges the reader's grasp of clinical theory and practice in an unexpected direction. Psychoanalysis in a New Key creates a deliberate focus on innovative and unsettling clinical thinking. Because that kind of thinking is encouraged by exploration of the sometimes surprising contributions to psychoanalysis of ideas and findings from other fields, Psychoanalysis in a New Key particularly encourages interdisciplinary studies. Books in the series have married psychoanalysis with dissociation, trauma theory, sociology, and criminology. The series is open to the consideration of studies examining the relationship between psychoanalysis and any other field—for instance, biology, literary and art criticism, philosophy, systems theory, anthropology, and political theory.

But innovation also takes place within the boundaries of psychoanalysis, and Psychoanalysis in a New Key, therefore, also presents work that reformulates thought and practice without leaving the precincts of the field. Books in the series focus, for example, on the significance of personal values in psychoanalytic practice, on the complex interrelationship between the analyst's clinical work and personal life, on the consequences for the clinical situation when patient and analyst are from different cultures, and on the need for psychoanalysts to accept the degree to which they knowingly satisfy their own wishes during treatment hours, often to the patient's detriment.

A full list of all titles in this series is available at:
https://www.routledge.com/Psychoanalysis-in-a-New-Key-Book-Series/book-series/LEAPNKBS

Reinventing Psychoanalysis for the Great Unknown

The Never-Ending Challenge

Ofra Eshel

with the collaboration of Charles Levin, Aner Govrin, Mary Tennes, Margaret Rubin, Ilan Bernat, and Dan Gilhooley.

Routledge
Taylor & Francis Group
LONDON AND NEW YORK

Designed cover image: The *Cat's Eye* nebula (NGC 6543). Credit: NASA, ESA, HEIC, and The Hubble Heritage Team (STScI/AURA)

First published 2027
by Routledge
4 Park Square, Milton Park, Abingdon, Oxon OX14 4RN

and by Routledge
605 Third Avenue, New York, NY 10158

Routledge is an imprint of the Taylor & Francis Group, an informa business

© 2027 Ofra Eshel

The right of Ofra Eshel to be identified as author of this work has been asserted in accordance with sections 77 and 78 of the Copyright, Designs and Patents Act 1988.

All rights reserved. No part of this book may be reprinted or reproduced or utilised in any form or by any electronic, mechanical, or other means, now known or hereafter invented, including photocopying and recording, or in any information storage or retrieval system, without permission in writing from the publishers.

For Product Safety Concerns and Information please contact our EU representative GPSR@taylorandfrancis.com. Taylor & Francis Verlag GmbH, Kaufingerstraße 24, 80331 München, Germany.

Trademark notice: Product or corporate names may be trademarks or registered trademarks, and are used only for identification and explanation without intent to infringe.

British Library Cataloguing-in-Publication Data
A catalogue record for this book is available from the British Library

ISBN: 9781041143642 (hbk)
ISBN: 9781041137313 (pbk)
ISBN: 9781003674078 (ebk)

DOI: 10.4324/9781003674078

Typeset in Times New Roman
by codeMantra

To my patients, my true partners in unknown ways.
With them I have learned—and am still learning—
the true meaning of delving into the heart of psychoanalysis.

Contents

About the author

Ofra Eshel is a clinical psychologist, training and supervising analyst, and senior faculty member of the Israel Psychoanalytic Society and Institute, and a Fellow of the International Psychoanalytic Association (IPA). She is also an honorary member of the New Center for Psychoanalysis, Los Angeles, and former vice president of the International Winnicott Association (IWA). She founded and heads the post-graduate track "Winnicott, Bion, and Independent Psychoanalysis: Radical Breakthroughs" at the advanced studies of the Program of Psychoanalytic Psychotherapy, Faculty of Medicine, Tel Aviv University, and (in 2024) the advanced program "Radical Breakthroughs in Contemporary Psychoanalysis" at Deepsprings, Beijing, China.

Her papers have been published in psychoanalytic journals and book chapters, translated into twelve languages, and presented at national and international conferences across four continents. She has been the recipient of several honors and awards, including a visiting scholar at PINC (San Francisco, 2013), the David Hammond grant at MIP (Boston, 2016), the Lecturer of the Psychoanalytic Center of California's 8th Annual Wilfred Bion Conference (Los Angeles, 2018), the 2021 Robert Stoller Lecture speaker (NCP, Los Angeles), and the Coralie Trotter Memorial Lecture (South Africa, 2025). She has been awarded the 2013 Frances Tustin International Memorial Prize and lecture, the 2017 Symonds Prize, and the 2022 Leonard J. Comess Award. In 2023, she was ranked as the first of the top 10 authors writing on Winnicott between 1978 and 2023. In 2012, she was featured in Globes (Israel's financial newspaper and magazine) as the sixteenth of the 50 most influential women in Israel. She co-edited *Was It or Was It Not? When Shadows of Sexual Abuse Emerge in Psychoanalytic Treatment* (2017) and authored *The Emergence of Analytic Oneness: Into the Heart of Psychoanalysis* (Routledge, 2019), translated into Chinese, Brazilian-Portuguese, and Hebrew, with Spanish and Russian translations currently in progress. She is in private practice in Tel Aviv, Israel.

Acknowledgments

This volume owes its becoming to the New Center for Psychoanalysis (NCP), Los Angeles, and the Leonard J. Comess Teaching Fund. It is based on the two-day conference *Reinventing Psychoanalysis for the Great Unknown—Ofra Eshel in LA*, held at the New Center for Psychoanalysis in March 2025. This was my fourth conference at NCP, following previous ones over the past 14 years—beginning in 2011, then in 2021, 2022, and 2025—during which I was also honored to deliver the 2021 Robert Stoller Memorial Lecture and to receive the 2022 Leonard J. Comess Award.

At these NCP conferences, I met the marvelous, internationally renowned discussants to whom I extend my heartfelt thanks: the late James Grotstein (2011), David Power (2021), João Carlos Braga, Ilan Bernat (2022), Charles Levin, Aner Govrin, Mary Tennes, and the clinical presenter Margaret Rubin (2025). The contributions of the last four—Charles Levin, Aner Govrin, Mary Tennes, and Margaret Rubin—at the 2025 conference are included in this volume. The Foreword by Ilan Bernat is also based on his presentation at the 2022 NCP conference. Together—along with the deeply evocative Afterthoughts by Dan Gilhooley—they form in this book, a rich and most illuminating tapestry of perspectives.

These welcoming NCP conferences, which allowed me the complete freedom to present and develop my own way of thinking, working, and writing—together with the unforgettable discussions and the responses from the audience—have opened for me further horizons of thought and feeling.

On a more personal note, I am profoundly grateful, first and foremost, to Dahlia Nissan Russ, chair of the Leonard J. Comess Teaching Fund, and to Tom Brod and Meiram Bendat, who joined her, for investing so much devotion in bringing these NCP conferences into being. I also extend my thanks to the NCP team and administration for their support. The 2025 conference was an especially difficult endeavor, held against the backdrop of massive traumatic events—the devastating fires in Los Angeles and the dreadful ongoing war in Israel.

I wish to thank wholeheartedly Donnel B. Stern, editor of the *Psychoanalysis in a New Key Book Series*, for his long-standing support over the years and for his immediate and warm encouragement of the idea of transforming the conference into a book. I am also grateful for the indispensable assistance of Kate Hawes and Aakriti Aggarwal in the making of this publication.

I have already expressed my profound indebtedness to my patients in the dedication to this book. I also wish to extend my many thanks to my colleagues and to the many candidates, supervisees, and students over the years at the Israel Psychoanalytic Society and Institute; the post-graduate track "Winnicott, Bion, and Independent Psychoanalysis: Radical Breakthroughs" in the Program of Psychoanalytic Psychotherapy, Faculty of Medicine, Tel Aviv University; the psychotherapy programs of Tel Aviv University and Bar Ilan University; my years-long Wednesday Reading Group; and the advanced program "Radical Breakthroughs in Contemporary Psychoanalysis" at Deepsprings, Beijing, China—where through the extraordinary help of Chen Ling (Linda), who translated my writings into Chinese, participants are able to read them in their own language. I would also like to add my deep gratitude to Dr. João Carlos Braga and Marina Vidal Stabile for graciously introducing my work to psychoanalysis in Brazil. With all of them, I have had—and continue to have—the opportunity to explore, think, discuss, and challenge theoretical and clinical ideas and questions while also thinking beyond what my own first-hand experience and reflections could have afforded me.

I owe special thanks to Lieske Bloom, who has assisted me with English editing over the years.

Lastly, and most significantly, I am profoundly grateful to my husband, Uzi—my loving, steadfast partner in every way—and to the heart-warming presence of our children Lee (and her partner Nadav) and Matan, my reliable helper with technical internet challenges.

List of contributors

Ilan Bernat, PhD, is a training and supervising analyst and faculty member at the Israel Psychoanalytic Society (IPS), and a Fellow of the International Psychoanalytic Association (IPA). He is a former director of the Training Committee of the Eitingon Institute, Israel Psychoanalytic Society. Dr. Bernat teaches seminars on Bion's work at the post-graduate track "Winnicott, Bion and Independent Psychoanalysis: Radical Breakthroughs" at the advanced studies of the Program of Psychoanalytic Psychotherapy, Faculty of Medicine, Tel Aviv University, and at the Israel Winnicott Center. He is in private practice for adults and adolescents in Kiryat Ono, Israel.

Ofra Eshel, PsyD, is a clinical psychologist, training and supervising analyst, and senior faculty member of the Israel Psychoanalytic Society and Institute, and a Fellow of the International Psychoanalytic Association (IPA). She is also an honorary member of the New Center for Psychoanalysis (NCP) in Los Angeles and former vice president of the International Winnicott Association (IWA). She founded and heads the post-graduate track "Winnicott, Bion, and Independent Psychoanalysis: Radical Breakthroughs" at the advanced studies of the Program of Psychoanalytic Psychotherapy, Faculty of Medicine, Tel Aviv University, and (in 2024) the advanced program "Radical Breakthroughs in Contemporary Psychoanalysis" at Deepsprings, Beijing, China. Her papers have been published in journals and books, translated into twelve languages, and presented at national and international conferences across four continents. She has been the recipient of several honors and awards. She has co-edited *Was It or Was It Not? When Shadows of Sexual Abuse Emerge in Psychoanalytic Treatment* (2017), and authored *The Emergence of*

Analytic Oneness (Routledge, 2019), translated into Chinese, Brazilian-Portuguese, and Hebrew, with Spanish and Russian translations in progress.

Dan Gilhooley, PsyaD, is a visual artist, psychoanalyst, and faculty member at the Center for Modern Psychoanalytic Studies (New York) and the Boston Graduate School of Psychoanalysis, where he teaches courses in research and comparative psychoanalysis and provides training analysis as well as clinical and research supervision. As a visual artist, he was elected to the National Academy of Design and has exhibited his drawings and paintings throughout the United States. In 2007, he was a research fellow in the IPA/Anna Freud Centre Psychoanalytic Research Training Program at Yale University. He has published psychoanalytic journal articles, authored book chapters, and presented papers at international conferences on the topics of psychoanalytic process research, intersubjectivity, creative imagination, and exceptional experience. His book, *Psychoanalysis, Intersubjective Writing, and a Postmaterialist Model of Mind: I Woke up Dead* (2020, Routledge), written with his patient Frank Toich, received a Gradiva Award for Best Psychoanalytic Book. In 2024 his paper "Dispelling illusions of locality: Panpsychism, telepathy, precognition, and modern psychoanalysis" won a Gradiva Award for best theoretical article.

Prof. Aner Govrin, PhD, is a clinical psychologist, philosopher, and psychoanalyst in private practice in Tel Aviv. He serves as director of the Psychoanalysis Hermeneutics doctoral program at Bar Ilan University's Program for Hermeneutics and Culture. A training analyst at the Tel Aviv Institute of Contemporary Psychoanalysis (TAICP), he co-founded the School of Psychoanalytic Psychotherapy at the Tel Aviv Institute and was its first director. He is the editor of the Routledge *Introductions to Contemporary Psychoanalysis* book series. His recent book, *How Philosophy Changed Psychoanalysis: From Naïve Realism to Postmodernism* (Routledge, 2024), explores the intersection of philosophical thought and psychoanalytic theory. His forthcoming work, *The Craft of Psychodynamic Case Study: Practical Guide*, will also be published by Routledge.

Charles Levin, PhD, FIPA, is a training and supervising analyst in private practice in Montreal and a Fellow of the IPA. He has served for many years in a variety of capacities at the Canadian Psychoanalytic Society and Institute, including director of training and editor-in-chief of the *Canadian Journal of Psychoanalysis*. In addition to clinical psychoanalysis, his work focuses on issues related to culture, aesthetics, and psychoanalytic ethics. His publications include *The Mind as an Internal Object* (Psychoanalytic Quarterly, 2010), *Art in the Offertorium: Narcissism, Psychoanalysis, and Cultural Metaphysics* (Rodopi, 2012), and the edited volume *Social Aspects of Sexual Boundary Trouble in Psychoanalysis*, which received an award from the APA Division 39 in 2021. He is currently completing a book-length study of Bion.

Margaret Rubin, PhD, is a member and senior faculty at the New Center for Psychoanalysis (NCP) in Los Angeles. She graduated from the Southern California Psychoanalytic Institute and Society in 2000 and was awarded Thesis of the Year. Additionally, she has twice been awarded Faculty of the Year at NCP for teaching relational theory to the psychoanalytic candidates in the training program. She has also taught in NCP's psychotherapy program. Dr. Rubin has published in *Contemporary Psychoanalysis* and *Psychoanalytic Dialogues*. She practices in Santa Monica, CA.

Mary Tennes, PhD, is a training and supervising analyst at the Psychoanalytic Institute of Northern California, where she is also faculty and the head of Faculty Development. In the last several decades, she has written and presented extensively on the intersection of psychoanalysis and the mystical, the telepathic, and the uncanny. Her most recent article, "Tell all the truth but tell it slant: Psychoanalysis and the uncanny," is about to be published in *Contemporary Psychoanalysis*. She is in private practice in Oakland, CA.

Credit list

I would like to thank the following journals and books for permission to be reprinted:

Rubin, M. (2025). Calamities and secrets, the power of the fetish. *Psychoanalytic Dialogues*, 35(2): 106–120. https://doi.org/10.1080/10481885.2025.2468703, publisher Taylor & Francis Ltd, https://www.tandfonline.com reprinted by permission of the publisher.

Eshel, O. (2025). Delving into the never-ending challenge of reinventing psychoanalysis for severe perversion. *Psychoanalytic Dialogues*, 35(2): 133–147. https://doi.org/10.1080/10481885.2025.2468721, reprinted by permission of Informa UK Limited, trading as Taylor & Francis Ltd https://www.tandfonline.com.

Eshel, O. (2025). Being totally in the dark: On working analytically within the depths of the Great Unknown of Psychic Catastrophe, pp. 82–103. In D. Power & D. Power (eds.), *The Somato-Psychic Realm*, Routledge. Copyright © 2025 by Imprint. Reproduced by permission of Taylor & Francis Group.

Section from:

Eshel, O. (2006). Where are you, my beloved? On absence, loss, and the enigma of telepathic dreams. *The International Journal of Psychoanalysis*, 87(6): 1603–1627. https://doi.org/10.1516/7GM3-MLDR-1W8K-LVLJ. copyright © 2006 Institute of Psychoanalysis, reprinted by permission of Informa UK Limited, trading Taylor & Francis Group, https://www.tandfonline.com on behalf of Institute of Psychoanalysis.

I am grateful for permission to use material from the following works:

From 'Wait for me and I'll come back!' by Konstantin Simonov (1941); translated by Avraham Shlonsky (1943). All rights are reserved to the author, Avraham Shlonsky, and ACUM.

From *My Michael* by Amos Oz, translated from the Hebrew by Nicolas de Lange in collaboration with the author. Copyright © 1968, Amos Oz, by Am Oved Publishers Ltd, used by permission of the Wylie Agency (UK) Limited. English Translation copyright © 1972 by Chatto & Windus Ltd and Alfred A. Knopf Inc. Reprinted by permission (United States and Canada) of Houghton Mifflin Harcourt Publishing Company. All rights reserved. Reproduced by permission (UK & Commonwealth) of The Random House Group Ltd. Copyright © 1972.

From "Poppies in October," Sylvia Plath. *The Collected Poems* by Sylvia Plath. Edited by Ted Hughes. Copyright © 1960, 1965, 1971, 1981, by the Estate of Sylvia Plath. Editorial material Copyright © 1981 by Ted Hughes. Reprinted by permission of HarperCollins Publishers. World permission granted by Faber and Faber Ltd.

From "East Coker" and "Little Gidding" from *Collected Poems 1909–1962* by T. S. Eliot. Copyright 1936 by Houghton Mifflin Harcourt Publishing Company. Copyright © renewed 1964 by Thomas Stearns Eliot. Reprinted by permission of Houghton Mifflin Harcourt Publishing Company. World permission granted by Faber and Faber Ltd.

From "A Dress of Fire," Dahlia Ravikovitch. *Collected Poems by Dahlia Ravikovitch*, 2010. Reprinted by permission of Hakibbutz Hameuchad Publishing, Tel Aviv.

Cover image: The *Cat's Eye* nebula (NGC 6543). Credit: NASA, ESA, HEIC, and The Hubble Heritage Team (STScI/AURA)

Foreword

'Blowing on the dying embers of a fire'[1]: Ofra Eshel's Promethean quest to expand the scope of psychoanalysis

Ilan Bernat

The publication of this volume, which explores the depth, originality, and far-reaching significance of Ofra Eshel's thought through her seminal lectures and the illuminating reflections of distinguished interlocutors, marks an important milestone in a long and fascinating journey. Throughout the three decades in which Eshel has engaged in psychoanalytic writing, her papers have been received by the psychoanalytic community with significant acclaim and esteem. Since 2019, which saw the publication of her first book to date, *The Emergence of Analytic Oneness: Into the Heart of Psychoanalysis*, Eshel has won even broader and more notable international recognition. Her distinction lies not only in being a prominent commentator on Winnicott and late Bion—and as one of the only authors to integrate the profound thinking of these two authors—but also in putting forth her own unique approach to clinical work with severe psychopathology and difficult treatment situations. Her work has been celebrated at many conferences and conventions worldwide. The two-day conference held at the New Center for Psychoanalysis in Los Angeles in 2025—"The Never-Ending Challenge of Reinventing Psychoanalysis for the Great Unknown"—on which this book is based, is proof of the deep interest and excitement with which her ideas have been received by notable authors. How does one account for such widespread interest? In what follows, I will attempt to outline some of the qualities of her thinking and writing that make her voice so compelling, innovative, and groundbreaking.

Eshel's singular voice on trauma

The philosopher Isaiah Berlin (1953) divides thinkers into hedgehogs and foxes, drawing inspiration for this distinction from the early Greek poet,

Archilochus, who argued that "a fox knows many things, but a hedgehog knows one big thing." Which category does Eshel belong to? Her erudition in psychoanalytic literature, nourished by her love for psychoanalysis and its pluralism, is both striking and rare. Still, deep down, she is without a doubt a veritable hedgehog. From her first steps as an analyst and a theoretician, she has devoted herself to 'one big thing': therapeutic presence. In her terms, this is 'presencing,'and the ensuing crucial and transformative unifying connection of two people, analyst and patient.

Eshel's writing has the urgent quality of a herald, seeking to awaken our awareness and transform the way we think about difficult patients, as well as others who risk being overlooked by psychoanalysis. I believe her voice, from the very beginning of her professional journey, has been a singularly intense and clear one within the psychoanalytic world. Over the years, she has shaped her own unique approach—what may be called "transformation in oneness"—inspired by her powerful, distinctive integration of Winnicott and the late Bion's thinking.

From where does this voice draw its force? I believe that, at its core, it stems not from her theoretical thinking nor from her vast clinical experience—though both play an important role—but from something deeper: a voice imprinted on her psyche. In her autobiographical paper (Eshel, 2010), she recounts a childhood overshadowed by profound family losses, bound up with the Holocaust and with the struggle to establish the state of Israel. She writes that

> We lived in an affluent neighborhood, in a house surrounded by trees, including a variety of fruit trees. There was a goldfish pond in front of our house, and an enormous Ficus tree that we and all the neighborhood children would climb and sit in for hours. We always had dogs and cats. But underneath, it all lay unspoken, concealed, unrecovered mourning, trauma, and a deep fear and trepidation of what life might bring.

She mentions the "agonizing years" that ensued after her uncle fell in the War of Independence, just one day before the declaration of the State of Israel:

> I was never able to participate, physically and emotionally, in Independence Day festivities. For years I tried to fathom this legendary, unknown uncle. I read his poetry and would gaze intently at the

> black-framed picture of him which, for years, had hung on our living room wall. His face was serious, stern, ascetic, and sincere. He was the uncle I longed to know.

Eshel's writing draws inspiration from these origins, where the catastrophes of kin she had never known live on within her psyche and become her own. Her attention to the unspoken, the absence, and the unrepresented pain that longs to be recognized and met—and begs to be deciphered—is a form of very early kind of attention. It reflects her personal memory, but also, to a significant extent, the collective memory of the history of Israel.

The 'hearing heart': ontological listening as the core of the therapeutic endeavor

The reader of Eshel's more recent papers will no doubt notice the intriguing fact that, while her clinical theory is constantly evolving and expanding, she often illustrates it using clinical material from her earlier practice. This offers the clear impression that, for Eshel, theory grows from the soil of clinical experience, rather than the other way around. Moreover, it shows how the clinical intuition that has guided her work from the very beginning had waited and evolved over many years within this depth of experiencing until it was elaborated and fully articulated into explicit theory. Eshel's clinical illustrations have a 'fractal-like' quality: each one encompasses elements that exist in others, making any clear distinction between her 'early' and 'late' work quite impossible.

The shared essence of these different illustrations involves, first and foremost, the way Eshel listens: her listening is patient and unrushed, attentive to the smallest details. It absorbs the full impact of her patients' presence and relentlessly seeks—together with them—to reach what has persistently withstood formulation and deciphering.

To get a sense of this unique form of listening, one may turn to her very first paper—"Story-telling in the analytic situation" (Eshel, 1996). This paper was written in Hebrew and has not been translated into English. It was written before Eshel began introducing her own language into the psychoanalytic vocabulary. In it, Eshel elaborates on her singular approach to analytic listening. She writes:

> In recent years, I find myself engaged in an almost inverse process regarding the stories told in treatment. From a suspicious, scrutinizing

> attitude – which fears that such stories seek to seduce, to avoid what really hurts, to distract from the analytic relationship – I have gradually learned to understand and listen to their potency, their meaning, their role, their emotional reverberation in myself and my patients. I have learned to attend the way in which the patient focuses and elucidates what is not understood, not expressed, not known, and accompany them on this journey. (p. 183)

Eshel sees great importance in listening to the centrality of the image for the patient as a therapeutic action that touches the patient's psyche in a deep yet non-invasive manner. In her view, what might seem like mere 'surface' actually touches on and joins together conscious layers with profound unconscious ones, establishing an analyst-patient connectedness. Eshel's listening begins by making room for the impressions that accumulate throughout the listening process, before applying any kind of conceptualization. I dub this way of listening *ontological listening.*

In the clinical illustration of this paper, one can palpably sense the extent to which Eshel views this kind of listening as a curative element in and of itself. She describes an eight-year-long analysis with a young man, who had difficulties expressing any kind of emotion or accepting any intervention that touched on emotion and relating. He talked in a truncated, disconnected, and withdrawn manner, and she "sat there for hours, trying to catch his fragmented, confused, disconnected words, trying to connect them and understand their meaning, sometimes understanding, and many other times not, becoming tired, paralyzed, fading out"—until he began to tell stories. The stories started out as the routine anecdotes and jokes he knew and would retell, which enabled him to connect with the world. But in analysis, the stories and jokes he told created a meeting place where he and Eshel could "live and experience together." These moments held an adequate distance for him wherein he was neither too detached nor too close, exposed, or penetrable. He could then be in touch with some inner content, feeling, fantasy, reflection, thought, and understanding from his inner living core, from his hidden true self. Within these stories, he responded keenly and sensitively to the treatment, in stark contrast to his other reactions. Over the years, remarkable changes unfolded in the patient's life, and in the analysis, his truncated speech turned into stories and dreams in which he was being saved and born, which ushered in the creation of a new selfhood. Interestingly, these changes do not appear essentially connected to interpretation.

In fact, Eshel does not mention a single interpretation throughout her entire account of the analysis.

At the end of the paper, Eshel offers a *personal note* on the "hearing heart," a biblical metaphor (I Kings 3:9) that first caught her attention as a young girl in primary school. She recalls her astonishment when reading about King Solomon, who asked God to give him a hearing heart to be able to judge his people. *How can a heart hear?* Eshel (2004, 2012, 2015, 2016a, 2016b, 2019a, 2019b, 2022a) would later develop this metaphor into one of the key ideas of her thinking. In my view, the "hearing heart" may be conceived as a notion that combines the ontological with the ethical.

Unlike her other conceptualizations, however, the "hearing heart" remains in that intermediary space between metaphor and formulated psychoanalytic concept, entailing a range of meanings that include heightened receptivity and being-with the patient's traumatic and unbearable parts. It also resonates with Freud's (1912) recommendation to the analyst that "he must turn his own unconscious like a receptive organ towards the transmitting unconscious of the patient" (p. 115). To this, Eshel (2019a) adds a special emphasis on heart-to-heart listening to heartbreak, "when the patient's communication is very broken and blocked." She thus underscores the analyst's need to open their heart, which can be understood as a plea for ontological, psycho-somatic listening, as opposed to mere hermeneutic listening.

Trauma, the ethical witness, withnessing and at-one-ment

In several of her recent articles from the past decade, Eshel (2016a, 2016c, 2019a, 2021, 2025) addresses the dream of the "burning child," described in chapter seven of Freud's *The Interpretation of Dreams* (1900, pp. 509–511). This dream was dreamed by a father who, after many days and nights of watching over his sick son, lost the boy. Exhausted, he lay down in the next room, leaving the door open so that he could still see into the room where his son's body was laid out, surrounded by tall candles, while an old man—hired to keep watch—sat murmuring prayers. Some hours later, the father dreamed that his son was standing beside his bed, grabbing him by the arm and whispering reproachfully, "Father, don't you see I'm burning?" The father woke up to a bright light coming from the next room. Rushing in, he saw that the old man had fallen asleep and that a candle had fallen over, burning the boy's shrouds and one of his arms.

At first, Freud interprets this dream as an instance of wish fulfillment: the dead child comes back to life for a moment, fulfilling the father's wish to see him alive once more, even if only briefly. Yet, Freud quickly rethinks this explanation, offering instead a different outlook:

> For it must be clearly understood that the easy and agreeable portion of our journey lies behind us. Hitherto, unless I am greatly mistaken, all the paths along which we have travelled have led us towards the light—towards elucidation and fuller understanding. But as soon as we endeavour to penetrate more deeply into the mental process involved in dreaming, every path will end in darkness.
>
> (pp. 510–511)

Eshel suggests that, in this passage, Freud is in fact returning to the trauma model he had abandoned three years earlier—a model that would re-emerge in his later theory of trauma in *Beyond the Pleasure Principle* (1920). Eshel seeks to retrieve this very trauma model, which she believes was relinquished all too soon.

Eshel also engages Lacan's reading of the dream, further developed by his student, the literary scholar Shoshana Felman, and Felman's student Cathy Caruth (1996). Referring to the same dream, Lacan (1973) introduced the notion of the trauma of the real into the process of dreaming itself. He noted that the child's question—"Father, don't you see I'm burning?" (Freud, 1900, p. 509)—has less to do with the father's wish to spend another moment with his child who had died and more to do with something else. In the dream, awareness chooses to remain asleep in the face of unbearable reality. This is symbolized by the figure of the old watchman, who fell asleep and failed to awaken even when the fire broke out. Here, it is *dissociation* rather than repression that severs the traumatic kernel (which had already been split off earlier, as the child grew ill and died) from the rest of the psyche.

The rebuking-pleading question of the burning child—"Father, don't you see I'm burning?"—echoes Jesus's heart-rending cry before his death: "My God, my God, why hast thou forsaken me?" (Matthew 27:46). Through father–son relations, the dream touches on the universal ethical order, as well as on our place, as clinicians, in the therapeutic ethical order. In contrast to the desire "to sleep," the voice of the survivor seeks to rouse us, to compel us to hear their story. For Lacan, the traumatic real demands an *ethical witness*.

The late psychoanalyst Dori Laub, who devoted himself to documenting the experiences of Holocaust survivors, writes in *Testimony*, which he co-authored with Felman (1992):

> The listener to the narrative of extreme human pain, of massive psychic trauma, faces a unique situation. [...] Massive trauma precludes its registration; [...] the trauma [...]—has not been truly witnessed yet, not been taken cognizance of. [...] The listener, therefore, is a party to the creation of knowledge *de novo* [...] By extension, the listener to trauma comes to be a participant and a co-owner of the traumatic event: through his very listening, he comes to partially experience trauma in himself.
>
> (p. 57)

Eshel further deepens this ethical-ontological thinking through what she calls 'withnessing,' a profound form of patient-analyst psychic interconnectedness, which even goes beyond intersubjectivity and strives for at-one-ment. To the discourse of witnessing trauma, she adds the psychoanalytic insight into infantile trauma—Winnicott's 'early breakdown' and the late Bion's 'mental catastrophe'—while emphasizing the element of analytic oneness in both theoreticians.

In Eshel's 'transformation in oneness' approach, withnessing and at-one-ment take precedence, to a great extent, over our conceptual psychoanalytic bread and butter: transference and counter-transference, the key role of interpretation, etc. This is an aspect of her approach that can easily be misunderstood. These key concepts are not done away with; rather, they are moved to the background while the deep ontological interconnectedness of two people creates a new force field of experience, in which me-you boundaries significantly dissolve. As Eshel (2019b) writes, "Patient and analyst 'live an experience together' (Winnicott, 1945) [...] or they live the unthinkable, the unexperienced, and the unlived t(w)ogether."

Two levels of transformations in oneness: the dialectics of reverie and at-one-ment

In her later works, Eshel (2022b, 2023, 2025) postulates two levels of transformation in oneness in the unrepressed unconscious that are determined by the depth of the trauma and the incapacity to represent, since representation is disrupted, regressively lost, or failed to develop. These two levels of transformation in oneness, inspired particularly by Winnicott's and Bion's radical late writings, open up new ontological–experiential possibilities for working within difficult psychic realities:

1. Transformation through withnessing or two-in-oneness, of 'partial or weak representation.'
2. Transformation through at-one-ment of what is 'unthinkable, unexperienced, unrepressed and unrepresented.'

Thus, these two different levels of depth partially or fully create transformation in oneness on various levels, as well as movement between these levels.

The phrase 'at one,' introduced as a psychoanalytic concept in the writings of the late Bion, has, according to the American Heritage Dictionary (2011), two meanings: to be in unity and to be in accord. Bion coined the term "at-one-ment," which refers to unity with the truth, with O (Lopez-Corvo, 2003), drawing inspiration from an existing word—'atonement,' which refers to reconciliation and accord between man and God. These two meanings of the phrase 'at one'—unity of emotional reality, O, and unity of relatedness—converge into a single multi-faceted experience. In my view, this experience exists at each of the levels of transformation in oneness as well as the reciprocal movement between them.

Eshel links the first level of transformation to the processes of 'the analyst's reverie, dream-thought, alpha function, and containing capacity'—and I view these aspects as entailing *both* above-mentioned meanings. This double meaning of unity increases and broadens the range of one's receptiveness to include subliminal messages from the patient, which are then transformed into α-elements (Bernat, 2022).

The second level of transformation, that of at-one-ment, is described by Eshel (2022) as often having a 'feeling of noetic revelatory quality,' as a 'quantum leap' which essentially changes the course of the treatment. It can be a moment or a process that lasts for more than a moment (Braga, 2021, 2022); in any case, it is more "unbidden" and less frequent than the first level of transformation.

Eshel makes a *unique* contribution through the radical formulation of this oneness, which is not easily grasped. Her view differs from other views, which emphasize the analyst's relation to themselves. Grotstein (2007), in discussing Bion's notion of 'becoming,' describes the analyst as

> receptive to his patient's emotional communications by being in exquisitely sensitive contact with *his own inner self* – that is, *his own*

> unconscious reservoir of *counterpart* emotions, experiences, phantasies, and so on, which match up with those of the patient.
>
> (p. 307; emphasis in original)

However, at a later time, Grotstein (2010) notes that, when working with "castaway patients," patients who have survived infantile catastrophes—in contrast with more healthy patients—this involves "the indivisibility of the transference <–> countertransference in the analyst's reverie, his or her capacity to '*become*' the analysand's anguish and agony." In these situations, he likens the analyst's experience to a "mystical religious rite of exorcism" (p. 25, italics in original).

Ofra is even more radical. When at-one-ment occurs, the analyst allows themselves to become completely immersed in the experience without acknowledging transference or counter-transference, or even without acknowledging their own exteriority in their role as analyst. This radical oneness is vital for effecting essential change in the therapeutic process and those taking part in it. However, this is not a state of fusion. The analyst is not *one* with the patient, but *at one* with them and their emotional reality (Eshel, personal communication, July, 2021).

The analyst's transformation

At a conference celebrating the publication of her 2019 book, held at the New Center of Psychoanalysis in Los Angeles, Eshel was asked the following question by her discussant, Dr. David Power (2021):

> I ask about it now, considering Ofra's work, because of the dread, the hopelessness, the despair and terror she asks herself to live through with her patients. Alongside the professional gratification of helping your patients, Ofra, do you find there's personal growth for you as well?

I will try to offer my own answer to this important question through the poem that Eshel (2021) cited in response: "A Dress of Fire" by the late Dahlia Ravikovitch (1969), one of Israel's most important women poets.

> Remember how Jason's wife burned in her dress?
> It was Medea, she said, Medea did that to her.
> You've got to be careful, she said....
> I said to her, ...
> I don't trust Greek tragedies.

But the dress, she said, the dress is on fire.
What are you saying, I shouted,
what are you saying?
I'm not wearing a dress at all,
this is me who is burning.

This poem stages a dialogue between two figures. The first is an observer who draws on her knowledge and recollection of the myth. While she warns of the impending disaster, her outlook is detached and blind to the poem's present reality. In contrast, the second figure—the one who is burning—speaks in the first person, desperately shouting out a terrible yet unacknowledged reality. Eshel uses this poem to illustrate a not-uncommon therapeutic pattern, in which the analyst/therapist's knowledge and insight serve to obscure a much more horrific reality that the therapist 'refuses' to see. However, the poem can also be read as entailing an ethic that enables the inner personal growth of those who practice it.

Literary scholar Giddon Ticotsky (2016) proposes reading the last line of the poem—"I'm not wearing a dress at all, / this is me who is burning"—as a moment of fundamental and unsettling self-revelation, which leads Ravikovitch to adopt an ethical stance of heightened sensitivity to, and responsibility for, the other (including a sense of social responsibility) in her later poems. The poem was inspired by an incident in the kibbutz children's society, in which she witnessed children catching a mouse and setting it on fire. The disaster of the other—the mouse—was transposed into the disaster of the speaker. Ticotsky links this movement in Ravikovitch to the ethical thinking of the philosopher Emmanuel Levinas. It is the transformation of trauma into ethical responsibility that connects Eshel to Ravikovitch's work and enables the analyst's personal growth.

Levinas (1961) describes this process as "desire burning with a fire that is not extinguished by saturation, thinking beyond what one thinks" (p. 33). Eshel's proposed transformation in oneness clearly resonates with Levinasian ethics and its enlivening fire. "To suffer the other," Levinas writes (1961), "is to take care of him, bear him, be in his place, consume oneself by him" (p. 64).

Levinas' ethical radicality, even more pronounced in his later writings (Levinas, 1974), entails a demand for maximal openness, for shedding one's defenses in the face of the other, passively exposing oneself, and avoiding any attempt to hold on to thematization—to the extent that one's self becomes fractured (Ben Pazi, 2012). This position turns into a being 'for the other,'

> burning for the other, consuming the bases of any position for oneself and any substantialization which would take form in this consummation, consuming even the ashes of this consummation, in which there would be a risk that everything be born again.
>
> (Levinas, 1974, p. 50)

Levinas' philosophical ethical radicality recalls Eshel's analytic ethical radicality. This is how Eshel (2016a, p. 85; 2019a, pp. 216–217) formulates the formidable challenge she sets before analysts and therapists:

> Thus, the critical question here, and in my opinion one of the most difficult questions at the heart of psychoanalytic work, is how willing are we—analysts and therapists—to reach to the unbearable realness of the patient's most traumatic experience, breakdown, and madness; to face the chilling horror and pain in hearing the voice that cries out from the bleeding wound; "a voice from the crypt" in Grotstein's (2010) words.

Indeed, this shared radicality entails a substantial risk of undermining the self of the analyst, but it also offers a unique boon. According to Levinas, this ethics grants the individual's subjectivity meaning and uniqueness, freeing them from the fixated clinging to sameness and familiarity.

A Promethean passion

In a seminar delivered in the last year of his life, Bion (1978, p. 46) said about difficult patients:

> We are presented with the debris, the vestiges of what was once a patient, and what still could be analogous to blowing on the dying embers of a fire, so that some spark communicates itself to others; the fire is built up again, although it appeared to be nothing but dead ash. Can we look at all this debris and detect in it some little spark of life?

The act of bringing the fire back into a person - into a patient whose soul was extinguished—may express a *Promethean passion*.

Psychoanalysis has generally been reserved, even reluctant, in addressing the figure of Prometheus, who stole fire from the gods to help mortals he pitied and was harshly punished for it. Some discussions portrayed him as driven by instinctual (Freud, 1932) or masochistic (Whitehead, 1987) desires. In contrast, Eshel—like Bion, Winnicott, and other groundbreaking psychoanalytic authors who have inspired her—has a burning, revolutionary psychoanalytic passion to expand the therapeutic scope to include those patients for whom psychoanalysis had not been able to make sufficient room for years. This ideal is often felt as defiant and rebellious and may indeed exact a price from its advocates. Neither of these perils has made Eshel's fire burn any less intensely.

Note

1 Bion, 1978.

References

American Heritage Dictionary of the English Language, 5th ed. In S. R. Kleinedler (ed.). New York: HarperCollins Publishers, 2011.

Ben Pazi, H. (2012). *Interpretation as an Ethical Act- Levinas' Hermeneutics.* Tel Aviv: Resling.

Berlin, I. (1953). *The Hedgehog and the Fox: An Essay on Tolstoy's View of History*. London: Phoenix, 2014.

Bernat, I. (2022). Negation as a method for intuiting psychoanalytic discoveries: Bion's turning point in "notes on memory and desire". In A. Grimalt (ed.), *Bion and Intuition in the Clinical Setting* (pp. 10–20). New York: Routledge.

Bion, W. R. (1978). The Tavistock seminars. In C. Mawson (ed.), *The Complete Work of W. R. Bion, Vol. IX*. London: Karnac, 2014.

Braga, J, C. (2021). Pathways to at-one-ment: Withnessing, receptivity and reverie. *IPA Congress*, June, 2021.

Braga, J, C. (2022). A different perspective on at-one-ment: Discussion of Ofra Eshel's "transformations on oneness". *São Paulo's Brazilian Psychoanalytic Society*, April, 2022.

Caruth, C. (1996). *Unclaimed Experience: Trauma, Narrative, and History*. Baltimore, MD & London: The Johns Hopkins University Press.

Eshel, O. (1996). Story-telling in the analytic situation. *Sihot-Dialogue, Israel Journal of Psychotherapy*, 10: 182–193.

Eshel, O. (2004). Let it be and become me: Notes on containing, identification, and the possibility of being. *Contemporary Psychoanalysis*, 40(3): 323–351.

Eshel, O. (2010). Patient–analyst interconnectedness: Personal notes on close encounters of a new dimension. *Psychoanalytic Inquiry*, 30(2): 146–154.

Eshel, O. (2012). In the dark depths "beyond the pleasure principle": On facing the unbearable traumatic experience in psychoanalytic work. *Sihot - Dialogue, Israel Journal of Psychiatry*, 27: 5–15.

Eshel, O. (2015). The "hearing heart" and the "voice" of breakdown. In L. Aron & L. Henik (eds.), *Answering a Question with a Question: Contemporary Psychoanalysis and Jewish Thought, Vol. II: A Tradition of Inquiry* (pp. 133–152). Boston, MA: Academic Studies Press.

Eshel, O. (2016a). The "voice" of breakdown: On facing the unbearable traumatic experience in psychoanalytic work. *Contemporary Psychoanalysis*, 52: 76–110.

Eshel, O. (2016b). The vanished last scream: Winnicott-Bion-Eigen. *IJP Open - Open Peer Review and Debate*, *3*: 1–32.

Eshel, O. (2016c). Psychoanalysis in trauma: On trauma and its traumatic history in psychoanalysis. *Psychoanalytic Review*, *103*: 619–642.

Eshel, O. (2019a). *The Emergence of Analytic Oneness: Into the Heart of Psychoanalysis*. London and New York: Routledge.

Eshel, O. (2019b). The vanished last scream: Winnicott and Bion. *Psychoanalytic Quarterly*, 88(1): 111–140.

Eshel, O. (2021). On a narrow bridge from soul to soul: Being there, being with, being at-one. *Sihot-Dialogue, Israel Journal of Psychotherapy*, 35: 238–251.

Eshel, O. (2022a). Bion's long road toward intuiting the patient's suffering: 'Theoretical' vs. 'clinical' Bion. *Contemporary Psychoanalysis*, 58: 46–76.

Eshel, O. (2022b). Being-in-oneness with the patient's experience – The analyst's struggle. Paper presented at online conference: *Transformations in Oneness in Psychoanalytic Work – A Day with Ofra Eshel*, New Centre for Psychoanalysis, Los Angeles, 5 February 22.

Eshel, O. (2023). When deadness breaks in: Surviving, "being-with" and a moment of "at-one- ment" in analytic work within deadness and emptiness. *Modern Psychoanalysis,* 47: 145–171.

Eshel, O. (2025). Delving into the never-ending challenge of reinventing psychoanalysis for severe perversion. *Psychoanalytic Dialogues*, 35: 133–147.

Freud, S. (1900). The Interpretation of dreams (second part). *SE*, 5: 339–626.

Freud, S. (1912). Recommendations to physicians practising psycho-analysis. *SE*, 12: 109–120.

Freud, S. (1920). Beyond the pleasure principle. *SE*, 18: 1–64.

Freud, S. (1932). The acquisition and control of fire. *SE*, 22: 183–194.

Grotstein, J. (2007). *A Beam of Intense Darkness- Wilfred Bion's Legacy to Psychoanalysis.* London: Karnac Books.

Grotstein, J. (2010). "Orphans of O": The negative therapeutic reaction and the longing for a childhood that never was. In J. V. Buren & S. Alhanati (eds.), *Primitive Mental States* (pp. 8–30). London: Routledge.

Lacan, J. (1973). *The Four Fundamental Concepts of Psycho-analysis*. Ed. J. A. Miller. London: Karnac Books, 2004.

Laub, D. (1992). Bearing witness, or the vicissitudes of listening. In S. Felman & D. Laub (eds.), *Testimony: Crises of Witnessing in Literature, Psychoanalysis, and History* (pp. 57–74). New York and London: Routledge.

Levinas, E. (1961). *Totality and Infinity: An Essay on Exteriority.* London: Springer, 2012.

Levinas, E. (1974). *Otherwise than Being, or Beyond Essence.* Pittsburgh: Duquesne University Press.

Lopez-Corvo, R. E. (2003). *The Dictionary of the Work of W.R. Bion.* London and New York: Routledge.

Power, D. (2021). At the frontier of analytic oneness: Presence, withnessing, and at-one-ment. Paper presented at the New Center for Psychoanalysis, Los Angeles, 24 January 2021.

Ravikovitch, D. (1969). *A Dress of Fire – Collected Poems by Dahlia Ravikovitch.* Tel Aviv: Hakibbutz Hameuchad Publishing, 2010. Also at: https://www.poetryinternational.com/en/poets-poems/poems/poem/103-3355_A-DRESS-OF-FIRE.

Ticotsky, G. (2016). *Dahlia Ravikovitch – In Life and Literature.* Haifa: University of Haifa Press & Miskal- Yedioth Ahronoth Books and Chemed Books.

Whitehead, C. C. (1987). On prometheus. *International Review of Psychoanalysis*, 14: 527–540.

Winnicott, D. W. (1945). Primitive emotional development. *International Journal of Psychoanalysis*, 26: 137–143.

Introduction

Where psychoanalysis dares the unknown: challenges and mysteries at the quantum frontier of psychoanalysis

Ofra Eshel

> Psychoanalysis goes far deeper than any other form of communication in a relationship that anybody knows so far. But … especially if we are going to have to deal with patients who are not really like the sort of patient spoken of in classical psychoanalysis, then not only are we to treat these patients, but we have to invent the methods by which we are going to treat them.
>
> (Bion, Los Angeles, 1967/2013)

The book gathers eight remarkably evocative presentations from the conference *Reinventing Psychoanalysis for the Great Unknown – Ofra Eshel in LA, 2025*, held at the New Center for Psychoanalysis, Los Angeles. Ofra Eshel's radical presentations are joined by discussions from internationally renowned psychoanalysts Charles Levin, Aner Govrin, and Mary Tennes; a deeply touching clinical case presentation by Margaret Rubin, discussed by Eshel and responded to by Rubin; and additional thought-provoking foreword and afterthoughts by Ilan Bernat and Dan Gilhooley. The decision to turn the conference into a book arose from the enthusiasm it inspired—born of the powerful combination of innovative theoretical material and moving clinical illustrations.

"Over the years," Eshel writes (2019), "I have come to think of extreme experiences in the clinical situation as a challenge to one's technique and complacent knowing. They evoke search and struggle, ingenuity and creative moves, at times leading us to extend, and even go beyond, the boundaries of our understanding and knowledge. They are an internal Rubicon that we have to cross." At the same time, encountering and writing about extreme experiences of the great unknown during treatment may be deeply puzzling, disturbing, sometimes mysterious, and always immensely difficult.

DOI: 10.4324/9781003674078-1

In her presentations here, Eshel ventures daringly into the essence of the great unknown in different realms of psychoanalysis: massively traumatic states, patients' enigmatic telepathic dreams, and the shattering sudden death of a patient. Moving beyond classical/conventional psychoanalysis and its epistemological boundaries, she explores the traumatic unknown and even the unknowable of catastrophic trauma—charting the ontological–experiential frontier of clinical work, which is of major and continuing revelatory quantum significance for her.

At the heart lies the critical idea that analytic oneness can open difficult-to-reach domains for further experiencing and transformation in treatment. Transformation is born within patient-analyst interconnected unknown. Patient-with-analyst, psyche-with-psyche, two-in-oneness (withnessing), or becoming at-one-with the patient's innermost traumatic reality may undergo the devastating experience that made it impossible for the patient to be there and experience it alone. Eshel believes that only by being within the patient's deep feeling states and their emotional impact can patient-with-analyst be given a new chance to relive and break through massive traumatic impacts.

The discussants of Eshel's papers highlight the profoundly creative and foundational quantum nature of her contributions—deeply inspired by the late Winnicott and Bion, yet reaching decisively beyond them.

As a whole, the book deepens theoretical and clinical understanding, opening both mind and heart to the dimension of radical presence and transformative experiential patient-analyst connectedness in analytic work. This offers new possibilities for extending the reach of psychoanalytic treatment and for working with some of the most difficult patients and treatment situations. At the same time, and no less importantly, it helps to withstand the unknown while building the capacity to contain and live through the ontological challenge of being and becoming in the experience—underscoring the significance of lived analytic oneness in this process.

The chapters in this book trace the unfolding of the conference—presentations followed by discussions, powerful, moving, and profoundly human—that take us into deep realms where the unknown, deep interconnectedness, and transformation meet.

Part I. Reinventing psychoanalysis for the great traumatic unknown introduces one of this book's core and critical themes—daring to enter the great unknown of unthinkable, catastrophic trauma and exploring what is genuinely possible within the analytic encounter with the unknown and the unthinkable.

This central clinical theme is first opened by Eshel's presentation in **Chapter 1, "Being totally in the dark: on working analytically within the depths of the great unknown of psychic catastrophe."** Eshel focuses, both theoretically and clinically, on the search, attempts, and struggle to reinvent psychoanalysis for working within the unknown and to extend the reach of psychoanalytic treatment into deep, non-communicating layers of the psyche. In Eshel's view, the essence of the great unknown in psychoanalysis is most deeply connected with massive traumatic states in which the patient's unbearable emotional reality becomes unthinkable, unexperienced, unrepresented, unknown, and inaccessible. This understanding draws particularly on Winnicott's and Bion's radical late writings—Winnicott on early unthinkable breakdown and Bion on mental catastrophe—along with Eshel's years of intensive clinical experience. Thus, the depths of the unknown, especially the most traumatic unknown, necessitate going beyond epistemological exploration to an ontological–experiential mode of work: *being and becoming* within the patient's unthinkable and unrepresented psychic reality—*psyche-with-psyche*—withnessing or becoming *at-one-with* the patient's innermost emotional reality. The unthinkable cannot be thought but only relived and gone through *with* the analyst.

The clinical example chosen to illustrate working within the grip of the great unknown is an extreme one: it describes the analyst's "sleep" during sessions—an unsettling, troubling, and rare phenomenon scarcely described in psychoanalytic literature. "I chose it," writes Eshel, "because it made me go through and face, more than any other clinical example I have written about, an experience that deeply puzzled me." Her recurring "sleep" during the sessions was approached as an open, central issue. In exploring this sleeping and its experiential qualities, Eshel foregrounds the analyst's being in the grip of a dissociative–dissociating process and the ensuing state of deep-level experiential patient-analyst interconnectedness/withnessing and their impact on each other. This line of thought engages with notions of the uncanny, dissociative self-states, and the transformation of the patient's dissociative self-experience through the analyst's vicarious dissociative experience.

Eshel's chapter is followed by two powerful **"Psychoanalytic wilderness with Ofra Eshel and her patient Clari," by Charles Levin,** grapples in a deeply thought-provoking way with the fundamental questions that Eshel's work raises about psychoanalysis as a form of treatment in deep layers of human experience and suffering. For Levin, Eshel's work reveals that while psychoanalytic learning, experience, and literacy are essential as preparation, there is, in the end, no fixed psychoanalytic technique available to us—except as a default position—especially in critical clinical situations. Eshel has addressed this disturbing reality in terms of the analyst's potential to "cross an internal Rubicon." What are the implications of this formulation for our professional identities as psychoanalysts? Can psychoanalysis integrate Eshel's deeply challenging insight into the contingency and precarity of our work?

In a manner that is unique in each case, Eshel intuitively discovers a point of contact with the patient beyond the "Rubicon," where analytic technique has ceased to function effectively. She immerses herself in the experiential reality of the relationship and allows herself to be carried forward with the patient in a singular process that cannot be adequately represented in conventional psychoanalytic terms.

Further, in her many writings on difficult and unusual case situations, Eshel encourages us to draw support particularly from Winnicott and Bion—a directive that is indeed helpful. Yet, it can be argued that her work points *beyond* the scope of these canonical psychoanalytic thinkers. Levin explains in detail how Eshel's way of working within the psychoanalytic setting differs in substantial ways from theirs.

For Levin, Eshel's practical understanding of psychic life resonates with the neurological–phenomenological model of the *embodied mind* as developed since the groundbreaking work of Varela et al. (2016). In a way that accords with her analytic mode of working, the phenomenological interpretation of current neuroscientific and neonatal research suggests that psychic life is an emergent property of the body in continuous interaction with others and with the physical and cultural environment. In that sense, the psyche is embodied, embedded, extended, and enactive within ecological and cultural space–time.

Eshel's riveting work suggests that the emotional reach of the psychoanalytic relationship can be extended into layers of human experience and suffering not yet sufficiently articulated by existing theory or technique. Levin frames her concept of "crossing the internal Rubicon" in terms of *surrendering* to the emotional logic of the inter-embodied mind and explores the implications of her clinical writings for psychoanalytic thought and practice.

The second discussion, **Chapter 3, "Fascinated and troubled in contemporary psychoanalysis: Ofra Eshel's extension of the Bion–Winnicott**

framework for working with severe traumatic states," by Aner Govrin, examines Ofra Eshel's distinctive contributions to psychoanalytic theory through his framework of "fascinated" and "troubled" psychoanalytic communities. He differentiates between two kinds of psychoanalytic communities that together sustain the development and resilience of psychoanalysis. *Fascinated* communities are characterized by loyalty to a single theoretical framework and a dedication to preserving and deepening its core ideas over time. *Troubled* communities, by contrast, adopt a critical stance, advocating for innovation and new theoretical directions in response to the perceived limitations of existing paradigms.

Govrin argues that the enduring tension and dialectic between these two modes of communities have enabled psychoanalysis to survive, adapt, and thrive despite both external criticism and internal crises. Within this framework, Ofra Eshel emerges as a "fascinated-troubled" analyst—deeply rooted in the Bion–Winnicott tradition yet working to innovate and transform it, particularly in addressing severe traumatic and catastrophic psychic realities.

Eshel's central contributions include the concepts of *Hinachechut* (presencing), analytic oneness, and the "hearing heart" and compassion, all of which highlight the analyst's ability and willingness to deep listening, emotional surrender, and compassionate *being-with* the patient in the most unthinkable and painful psychic territories. Her approach moves beyond interpretation and containment, advancing an ontological presence and a compassion that means "to suffer-with" as the very core of clinical work.

Eshel's innovations fill gaps in classical theory, particularly in working with "unthinkable" or unrepresented realms of traumatization, and they offer a comprehensive clinical framework for working with patients in deep psychic darkness. Govrin concludes that these innovations arose from clinical necessity—from Eshel's unwavering commitment to reach seemingly unreachable patients and to transform their most unknown traumatic states. Through her work, Eshel exemplifies how the creative balance between loyalty and disruption continues to propel psychoanalytic thought and practice forward.

Part II. The enigma of telepathic dreams ventures into the unknown of the profound mystery of telepathy in psychoanalysis. Telepathy—*suffering (or intense feeling) at a distance* (from the Greek *pathos* + *tele*)—refers to the transfer or communication of thoughts, impressions, or information between two people without the use of the recognized sense organs. It is a realm from which psychoanalysis has, over the years, largely turned away in trepidation. Dream telepathy (especially patients' telepathic dreams) and related telepathic phenomena within the psychoanalytic context have been a controversial and disturbing "foreign body" ever since telepathy was introduced into psychoanalysis by Freud in 1921.

In **Chapter 4—"Where are you, my beloved? On absence, loss, and the enigma of telepathic dreams,"** Ofra Eshel explores this profound enigma through her analytic encounters over the years with telepathic dreams of five patients—dreams containing precise details of the time, place, sensory impressions, and experiential states that the analyst was in at that time—details the patients could not have known through ordinary sensory perception or communication.

Eshel's ensuing explanation combines three contributory factors: the patient, archaic communication, and the analyst. In each of these patients, the mother during early childhood was emotionally absent, mostly absent-within-absence; that is, a mother physically present yet emotionally absent from her child's early life, often due to the absence of a significant figure in her own life. This condition fostered a fixation on a nonverbal, archaic mode of communication. The patients' telepathic dreams, Eshel suggests, are formed to serve as a psychic search engine—to find the analyst when he or she is suddenly emotionally absent, and thus to halt the process of abandonment and prevent a collapse into the despair of the early traumatization.

In this way, the telepathic dream embodies an enigmatic "impossible" extreme of deep-level patient-analyst *quantum interconnectedness* and unconscious communication within the analytic process.

In **Chapter 5—"To approach what is radically other,"** Mary Tennes, in her evocative discussion, extends these questions. Telepathic phenomena within psychoanalysis challenge our established notions of time, space, and selfhood. The analytic capacity to open to—and to be altered by—that which disrupts our ordinary sense of self is beautifully exemplified in Eshel's sensitive clinical approach.

Tennes suggests a distinction between exploring the function of telepathic dreams within a given analysis and attempting to explain the awe-inspiring, disruptive realities they present. She also proposes that the willingness to recognize an inexplicable interconnectedness between self and other—resonant with findings in contemporary physics—bears profound relevance to our capacity to address current global catastrophes.

Part III. Reinventing psychoanalysis for severe perversion centers on the clinical illustration of the analytic treatment of a severely fetishistic patient, presented in **Chapter 6—"Calamities and secrets, the power of the fetish: clinical case,"** by Margaret Rubin. Rubin examines the developmental consequences of a fractured self, maintained and held together by physical restraints that, over time, morphed into an unusual fetish dominating the patient's life. Although initially lifesaving by giving him the illusion of power over his tormentors—primarily his psychotic mother whose unleashed, manic sexual behaviors had inscribed themselves upon his mind and body—his fetish kept him embedded in a fixed and repetitive pattern of living in a frozen past that obfuscated the possibilities of a living future. Over fits and starts to his seven-year analysis, the patient was able to gradually leave the safety of his universe of one for the unpredictability of the relational world—no small feat given the enactment that almost ended his treatment. The patient's split-off affective experiences were accessed through the medium of his remarkable dreams. As the relationship with his analyst deepened, he was able to open himself to the present and to hope for a changing future.

The treatment was abruptly terminated by the patient's sudden death.

In **Chapter 7, "Delving into the never-ending challenge of reinventing psychoanalysis for severe perversion,"** Ofra Eshel offers a comprehensive discussion of Rubin's case. For Eshel, the discussion of Rubin's clinical case becomes an invitation to dive into the long-standing challenge of reinventing psychoanalysis for severe perversion—and, more broadly, into the challenge of extending the reach of psychoanalytic treatment to more disturbed patients and traumatic states of mind, a theme woven throughout this book.

Her discussion draws on her clinical analytic experience with severe cases of sexual perversion she has treated over the years and is inspired primarily by Winnicott's radical late writings on early breakdown and Grand's description of "catastrophic loneliness."[1]

Eshel emphasizes, even more so in the treatment of perversion, the new theoretical-clinical possibilities that come into being through the analyst's abiding presence and the ensuing deep patient-analyst interconnectedness, which together forge the fundamental ontological–experiential dimension of analytic work, with its quantum essence. Because of the dissociative, secretive nature of perversion, because of it being a self-induced survival solution through dissociative splitting and a compulsively driven and exciting ritual that does not truly change the deep inner stalemate—the pervert cannot be extricated from these repetitive cycles alone. Hence, Eshel focuses on the unique challenges faced by analysts/therapists in going beyond epistemological (knowing) exploration and interpretation to *being and becoming in the experience*, interconnected with the patient's psychic reality. The critical idea, as emphasized throughout this book, is that by being within the patient's deeply unbearable states, patient-with-analyst are given a new chance to relive and break through massive traumatic impacts and catastrophic loneliness.

Finally, in addressing the patient's death in the analysis, Eshel reflects on the dangers inherent in this psychoanalytic work of reaching into and activating catastrophic depths of psychic traumatization—so that the change of deadness-aliveness in treatment is radical and perilous. Part III concludes with **Chapter 8—"Bearing the unbearable,"** Margaret Rubin's poignant and deeply personal response to Eshel's discussion: "Dr. Eshel's profoundly rich commentary brought my patient back to me in high relief. I am grateful for her deep understanding of his fetish and his subsequent struggles in managing what she refers to as the distortion of life's fundamental processes of relatedness. Her suggestion that his addiction was not to the belt but to me—to the treatment—had been overlooked. Although I understood the clinical necessity of his regression to dependence, I was uncertain if I could hold and contain his fears and emerging needs that had been safeguarded by my protective presence. I, too, had to surrender to this process—a daunting proposition, as there is no 'how to do' this. I believe my fear of failing him contributed to my dissociating from how necessary I was to his going on being. Eshel's examination of 'too much aliveness' resonated deeply with me. Both of these ideas are discussed in my response to her commentary."

This book is greatly enriched with a most beautiful **Foreword** and **Afterthoughts,** each opening further horizons of thought and feeling.

Ilan Bernat's foreword is based on his discussion at an earlier 2022 conference in Los Angeles honoring Ofra Eshel. The **Foreword, *"Blowing on the dying embers of a fire*[2] *: Ofra Eshel's Promethean quest to expand the scope of psychoanalysis*,"** traces the essential qualities of Eshel's three decades of psychoanalytic writing, highlighting—theoretically, clinically, and personally—what makes her voice so innovative and groundbreaking.

Writing with the urgency of a herald, Eshel seeks to awaken analytic awareness and to transform how we think and work with our most difficult patients. Her concept of *transformation in oneness* offers a radical ontological listening—a "hearing heart" that absorbs the impact of the patient's presence before any conceptualization, joining the *ontological with the ethical* in a heart-to-heart attunement to heartbreak.

In her rereading of Freud's "burning child" dream, Eshel expands the notion of witnessing trauma into *withnessing*—a profound psychic interconnectedness that transcends intersubjectivity and aspires toward at-one-ment. For Eshel, these modes of being take precedence over interpretation, transference, or counter-transference, long considered the core of psychoanalytic work.

Further developing her radical approach, she postulates two levels of transformation within the *unrepressed unconscious*: transformation through *withnessing* or "two-in-oneness" of partially represented experience, and transformation through *at-one-ment* of what is unthinkable and unrepresented. These processes dissolve epistemological boundaries while creating new unifying relations, corresponding to the dual meaning of "at one": emotional unity and relational unity. The analyst must risk total immersion to bring about essential change.

Eshel's vision also transforms the analyst. Drawing on Eshel's citation of Dahlia Ravikovitch's *A Dress of Fire*, Bernat links the motif of burning to the burning for the other in Levinas's ethics of responsibility, where exposure to the other's suffering threatens the analyst's self, yet gives rise to new meaning and uniqueness.

For Bernat, like Bion, Winnicott, and other groundbreaking psychoanalytic thinkers who inspired her, Eshel carries a burning, revolutionary Promethean passion to widen the therapeutic field for those patients to whom psychoanalysis had long struggled to offer space and hope. It is precisely this ethical fire that renders her voice so vivid and so compelling today.

Dan Gilhooley's **Afterthoughts**, ***"The generative power of living-through death in the work of Ofra Eshel,"*** concludes the book with remarkable depth and power. Ofra Eshel—he writes—is a masterful clinician working at exceptional depth. Within a Winnicottian model of deep shared regression, she reaches back emotionally with her patient to a moment of early traumatic breakdown—when the patient psychically confronted extinction that damaged them. There, drawing on Bion's conception of *transformation in O*, Ofra becomes the patient's psychic reality, living-through the catastrophic experience of annihilation while remaining alive. Through their state of at-one-ment, the patient rises from psychic death—like Lazarus. This transformation in oneness restores life from psychic death and lies at the heart of Eshel's clinical genius.

Regressions to moments of annihilation propel analysts back to the unknown origins of mind—or to birth itself, that primal struggle of life and death. In this realm of "pre-existence," eschewing the security of the already known, Ofra pursues the great unknown—even the unknowable. Encountering "impossible" and mysterious telepathic experiences with her patients and working intuitively and totally in the dark, she is guided by her deep faith in the unconscious psychoanalytic process.

From this threshold invitation of the Introduction, let us move into the chapters that follow—where, in the living encounter, psychoanalysis meets and is met by the unknown.

Notes

1 Grand, 2000.
2 Bion, 1978.

References

Bion, W. R. (1978). The Tavistock seminars. In C. Mawson (ed.), *The Complete Work of W. R. Bion, Vol. IX*. London: Karnac, 2014.

Grand, S. (2000). *The Reproduction of Evil*. Hillsdale, NJ: Analytic Press.

Varela, F., Thompson, E. & Rosch, E. (2016). *The Embodied Mind: Cognitive Science and Human Experience.* Revised Edition. Cambridge, MA: MIT Press. (Originally published 1991).

Part I

Reinventing psychoanalysis for the great traumatic unknown

Chapter 1

Being totally in the dark

On working analytically within the depths of the great unknown of psychic catastrophe

Ofra Eshel

Introduction

Contemporary psychoanalytic approaches strive to extend the reach of psychoanalytic treatment and to reinvent psychoanalysis for the great unknown—which, in my view, has become primarily connected to massive traumatic unknown, and even the unknowable of catastrophic trauma and breakdown. Over the past decades, psychoanalytic thinking has moved theoretically and clinically into the traumatic depths of human experience—both personal and collective, direct or transmitted across generations—and toward an increased emphasis on the distortion of fundamental processes of relatedness. This has called for changes in psychoanalytic thinking and technique. Working psychoanalytically with non-neurotic patients and traumatized states of mind challenges traditional theory and practice and, to my mind, opens a new dimension of essential presence and transformative experiential patient-analyst connection—one that twenty-first-century psychoanalysis is not only moving toward but must also deepen into if it is to meet its clinical challenges alongside the emerging possibilities.

This move resonates with the ontological shift that is taking place in psychoanalysis (Eshel, 2004, 2017, 2019a; Ogden, 2019), which reflects a fundamental commitment to the principle of *being and becoming in the experience* rather than an epistemological exploration and interpretation.

Being-within, being-with, being-at-one-with: on transformations in oneness

At this transformative juncture, critical and challenging clinical questions arise: *Can analytic work reach the great unknown of unthinkable catastrophic trauma? What is genuinely possible within the analytic encounter with the unknown and the unthinkable?*

DOI: 10.4324/9781003674078-3

My own way of thinking and working analytically—and of engaging with these pressing questions—has, over the years, turned toward the ontological-experiential possibilities inherent in analytic work. Based on my clinical experience, this has forged and delineated an *ontological-experiential dimension* that has become, for me, a fundamental dimension of clinical psychoanalysis. It has centered on two key terms: the analyst/therapist's "*presencing*" (being-there) within the patient's experiential psychic reality and the grip of the analytic process, and the ensuing deep patient-analyst interconnectedness or "withnessing"—an emergent new entity of patient-with-analyst, *a two-in-oneness,* that may deepen into *at-one-ment* with the patient's innermost emotional reality; a living entity that is fundamentally inseparable into its two participants. Analyst and patient are inevitably bound together through this way of analytic work. This is primarily an *interconnected* relatedness rather than an interactive relationship, and it concentrates on the *ontological (being) quality* of the analytic experience that is lived through *with* the analyst rather than the epistemological (knowing) and interpretive qualities. The analyst gives himself over to becoming part of the patient's ongoing emotional reality and mental processes as an area of receptivity, experiencing, processing, and transformation. Patient-and-analyst "live an experience together" (Winnicott, 1945, p. 152, italics in original; see also Ogden, 2001), or they "live the unthinkable, the unexperienced, and the unlived t(w)ogether" in living through extremely dark, unknown processes in difficult treatments (Eshel, 2019b). This patient-analyst entity of experiencing and be(com)ing in-oneness allows for traumatic experiences that the patient has been unable to bear, to enter the now and be jointly met, experienced, and lived through t(w)ogether.

I have also called this process in its extreme singularity "quantum interconnectedness" (from physicist David Bohm's [1980] phrase "the quantum interconnectedness of distant systems"), in order to convey the profound implications of this quantum-like psychoanalytic quality of experience.[1]

The spectrum of analytic oneness

This ontological-experiential way of working is a fundamental dimension of my analytic work with patients. But varying states of the unknown or unthought intensify and develop into the full need and the full potential of the ways of being, becoming, and experiencing-in-oneness in the analytic work; namely, the *analytic oneness* as an essential resource for the process of transformation.

In recent years, particularly inspired by Winnicott's and Bion's radical late writings along with my clinical experience, I have formulated and mapped a **spectrum of analytic oneness**—a spectrum of varying degrees of patient-analyst oneness and transformations in oneness when working within different unconscious or unknown states and non-communicating layers in the analytic work. It focuses primarily on the extent of the traumatization or the distortion of fundamental processes of relatedness, and the incapacity to represent, since representation is disrupted, regressively lost, or failed to develop. At the same time, it opens up new ontological-experiential (rather than epistemological) possibilities for working within difficult psychic realities, through the analyst/therapist presencing and patient-analyst being and becoming-in-oneness. It also further investigates the meaning of going beyond the limits of representations and epistemological exploration, toward ontological-experiential, quantum work within the unthinkable and unrepresented.

The spectrum includes:

1. At one end of the spectrum is **The Freudian repressed unconscious**—consists of psychic material that could be repressed, in which "the interpretation of dreams is the royal road to a knowledge of the unconscious activities of the mind" (Freud, 1900, p. 608, italics in original); Namely, an epistemological exploration for the recovering of repressed intrapsychic material through the interpretation and analysis of the transference and the interpretation of dreams. This is the most differentiated mode of analytic functioning.

   However, despite the centrality of the Freudian repressed unconscious, Freud himself (1915, 1923) pointed out that although what is repressed is unconscious, the unconscious is not only the repressed:

   > We recognize that the *Ucs.* does not coincide with the repressed; it is still true that all that is repressed is *Ucs.*, but not all that is *Ucs.* is repressed. .... [W]e find ourselves thus confronted by the necessity of postulating a third *Ucs.*, which is not repressed.
   >
   > (1923, p. 18, italics in the original)

2. **The unrepressed unconscious** of non-neurotic patients and states of mind consists of psychic material that could not be repressed, but is dissociated, split off, and may become unrepresented (Levine et al., 2013; Vermote, 2013; Bergstein, 2014; Eshel, 2017, 2019a; Levine, 2022). Thus, the unconscious in the realms of unbearable and catastrophic psychic trauma is no longer the repressed unconscious of psychoneurosis. It is the unrepressed unconscious, and it attempts to extend psychoanalytic practice beyond psychoneurosis and beyond what were formerly thought to be the limits of analytic work. Taking this further (Eshel, 2021, 2023, 2025a,b, 2026), it ranges from the unrepressed realm, *level **I***, that is traumatically dissociated and unknown, to the deeper unrepressed and unrepresented realm, *level **II***, of pre-mental states of primordial beingness, and, particularly, the most unknown and unknowable, unthinkable traumatic psychic reality; the deepest traumatic and non-communicating issues of human life.

Analytic work in the unrepressed unconscious entails being in various degrees of patient-and-analyst state of oneness and transformations in oneness, moving from patient-and-analyst *two-in-oneness* (level **I**) to *at-one-ment* with the patient's unrepressed and unrepresented psychic reality (level **II**):

Level I. The unbearable traumatic unknown remains at the level of partial or weak representations—"Was it or was it not" and "shadows" of remembering (Eshel & Zeligman, 2017), sometimes driven to the verge of the unrepresented. This dissociated, traumatically unknown is received by the analyst, and can be processed and transformed in different ways of psychic functioning: by analytic representations through the analyst's reverie, dream-thought, alpha function, containing capacity—in Bionian, intersubjective and analytic field models inspired by Bion's earlier, projective/introjective identification model (1959, 1962); by patient-and-analyst's interactional states of being and experiencing in the interpersonal and relational field and enactments (Bromberg, 2006, 2011; Stern, 2015, 2019); by "vicarious introspection" in Kohut's (1984) Self-psychology; by Botella & Botella's "The Work of Figurability," and the analyst's "working as a double" (2005); by de M'Uzan (2006) "psychological chimera" that emanates from the unconscious minds of the analysand and analyst; and more. These are "transformations in K" (Bion, 1965, 1970; Vermote, 2013), thus getting to *know* and transforming together, even as one mind dissociates, through *patient-with-analyst two-in-oneness.* Many of the contemporary psychoanalytic concepts of analytic work belong to this level **I**.

Level II. But in the unfathomable and unthinkable realm—of pre-mental states of primordial human beingness, the unknown and unknowable origins of the personality; and, especially, the darkest depths of traumatization, in particular the great unknown of mental catastrophe (Bion, 1970) and early breakdown (Winnicott, 1974/1963, 1965)—the patient's abysmal emotional reality is mostly unthinkable, unexperienced, unrepressed and unrepresented because it was so unbearably dreadful that it could not be experienced and thought at the time. This necessitates going *beyond* the limits of representations and analytic thinking, dreaming and containing (K) to a mode of *being*—to the ontological-experiential analytic work of being-there (presencing), within the darkness of the innermost traumatic psychic reality, becoming at-one-with[2] the patient's abysmal emotional reality of the great unknown. It is "the analyst's intuitive contact with the emotional situation itself" (Bion, 1965, p. 76), "the thing itself, the fundamental reality" (2013, p. 3), by becoming at-one-with it, which is at the core of the clinical work. This way is essentially other than to seek for what can be thought, known, and interpreted. *The unthinkable cannot be thought, but only relived and gone through with or at-one-with the analyst.*

In Bion's powerful words:

> This means that the understanding of the patient and the identification with him that have been regarded as sufficient hitherto must be replaced by *something quite different*. The transformation in K must be replaced by the transformation in O, and K must be replaced by F[aith]... by the suspension of memory, desire, understanding ... It must be a science of at-one-ment. It must have a mathematics of at-one-ment, not identification ... With this [O] he [the psychoanalyst] must be at one.
>
> (Bion, 1970, pp. 45–46, 89, my italics)

Namely, suspending attention to the already known, and *becoming at-one* with the innermost emotional unknown, unthinkable, and inaccessible of the patient or the session.

And in Winnicott's different, uniquely evocative style, at the end of his life, on this very point: "I am asking for a kind of revolution in our work. Let us re-examine what we do. It may be that in dealing with the repressed unconscious we are colluding with the patient and the established defences" ("DWW's Notes for the Vienna Congress, 1971" that were never presented because of his untimely death; cited by Abram, 2013, pp. 1, 312).

> [S]omething fundamental had remained unchanged … my interpretations, made on good grounds … -- why such interpretations were never mutative. They were accepted, but: so what? Now that *the new position* had been reached the patient felt a sense of relationship with me, and this was extremely vivid. It had to do with identity. The … split-off element found *a primary unity with me* as analyst, and this gave the man *a feeling of having started to live* ... For my part, I have needed to live through a deep personal experience in order to arrive at the understanding I feel I now have reached.
>
> (Winnicott, 1971, pp. 90, 86, my italics)

Namely, *primary unity* rather than epistemological-interpretative exploration is crucial in the most traumatic and split-off domains.

The becoming of at-one-ment is an ontological *quantum leap* in psychoanalytic thinking and practice. The analyst-at-one-with-patient is given a radical new chance to reach and experience the patient's most traumatic, unthinkable, and unrepresented, non-communicating emotional reality in a deep, new sense of to be and to understand it. From here on, the treatment process is changed in some essential way. All that belongs to knowledge comes to us through this at-one-ment and the subsequent transformation (evolution) of this state. This and only this will be accounted for in the interpretation (Bion, 1970; Green, 1973; Braga, 2021, 2022).

To sum up: Ferro (2021) highlights "the transition [in psychoanalysis] from a theory and technique based on interpretation to a theory and technique whose pillars are transformations" (p. xvii). I further point out that transformations entail *transformations in oneness*; namely, varying patient-and-analyst states of oneness which come to life in the analytic work, moving from patient-and-analyst *two-in-oneness* to *at-one-ment* with the patient's deepest traumatic, non-communicating emotional reality. I would say, paraphrasing Meltzer (1967) on the analytic process, that the analyst at work must be "lost" in the depths of analytic oneness, trusting in the virtuosity of his or her psyche within these experiences of absorption. *The critical idea is that analytic oneness can open difficult-to-reach domains for further experiencing and transformation in treatment.* Patient-with-analyst or patient-at-one-with-analyst, psyche-with-psyche, may undergo the devastating experience that made it impossible for the patient to be there and experience it alone.

I believe that only by *being within* the patient's deep feeling states and their emotional impact, can patient-with-analyst be given a new, transformative experiential chance to relive and break through massive traumatic impacts. The catastrophic impact turns into a *catastrophic change* (Bion, 1965) and can become-with the analyst a *catastrophic chance.* Patient-with-analyst are given a new chance to live it.

In T. S. Eliot's powerful words:

> Into another intensity
> For a further union, a deeper communion
> Through the dark cold and the empty desolation…
>
> (*East Coker*, p. 204)

In the grip of the unknown

From this broader and theoretical introductory context, I will proceed to the crucial subject of this presentation—Working analytically within the depths of the great unknown of psychic catastrophe, "in the grip of the process" (Searles, 1965, p. 36).

The clinical example that I have chosen to illustrate the work of being and becoming within the patient's unknown realms of emotional catastrophe is an extreme example (earlier versions published in 2001, 2019a). It describes my experience of sleeping during treatment. I chose it because this treatment made me go through and face, more so than any other clinical example that I have written about, an experience that deeply puzzled me. When I first wrote about it (Eshel, IJP, 2001), I focused primarily on the subject of the analyst's 'sleep.' I reviewed the psychoanalytic literature on the analyst's sleeping during sessions, and then focused on exploring my own sleeping and its qualities of experience while also relating to the deliberation over self-exposure and concealment of such difficult experiences. Later, in my book (2019a), I added in this regard Bion's (2005) powerful words in his sixth Rome seminar (on 16 July 1977—Morning), at the age of eighty:

> It seems to me that the analyst who actually participates in the experience has a chance of deciding whether to try to communicate, and whether we would be capable of hearing and understanding the communication. If he is to communicate the experience, which language is he to talk? Will articulate speech do? … In any case it requires courage if he is going to dare to make public, to communicate to somebody not himself, his experience. It may take a long time.
>
> (p. 64)

In the present article, I will focus mainly on the darkness and working totally in the dark, which resonates with Francesca Bion's description that Bion "often talked to her about his feelings of *being totally in the dark* … He would say, … 'It's beyond me,' or, 'I can't make head or tail of it'" (1995/2014, p. 96, my italics). These words strongly relate to moments of my own inability to understand during that analytic process.

I will first let the clinical material speak, describing a clinical sequence in which the extreme unknown during the sessions became an open issue, and closely follow my experience of being in the grip of this process as the treatment unfolded. I will then return to this dark unknown in the discussion, in an attempt to rethink and understand it more fully.

Clinical illustration

Background

Clari came to me unwillingly for treatment after undergoing two years of twice-weekly face-to-face therapy with a female psychotherapist to whom she had become considerably attached. Clari, then in her early 30s, was born in South America, and was the second of three daughters born at three-year intervals. Her younger sister had been very ill from the age of six months. She was kept alive for nine years, in a permanent "vegetable" state, until her death when Clari was twelve years old, two years after the family immigrated to Israel, leaving the child behind in an institution. Clari married at 20, but her relationship with her husband was difficult and sexually frightening. She left him and, for nine years, lived with a woman in a stable but stagnant relationship dominated by her partner's obsessive-compulsive preoccupations. She originally sought therapy because of severe anxiety attacks during a period of war in Israel. The therapy was warm and supportive, in the best sense of the word, and led to a turnabout in her life: she decided she wanted to have children but thought that children should grow up with a mother and a father. She therefore decided to leave the woman with whom she had been living and establish a relationship with a man.

It was at this point that Clari's psychotherapist was informed that, unexpectedly, she would be leaving Israel within a few months for family reasons. Therefore, she asked me to accept Clari for treatment, as she was concerned about abandoning her at such a stage of critical decision-making. I was unable to accept Clari then, since I had no vacancy, and suggested referring her to another therapist, but Clari's psychotherapist pressed me to take her because she felt I was strong enough to treat Clari during this angry, stormy time. I finally agreed, on the condition that the treatment begin in six months' time.

Before committing ourselves to treatment, Clari and I met once, at her suggestion. During that session, she expressed a reluctant and rejecting attitude toward me, glancing suspiciously at the couch—even though she would be coming for twice-weekly face-to-face therapy, as in the therapy she had been undergoing—saying that she would never have gone to a psychoanalyst for treatment, and the only reason that she came was because her therapist had recommended me so warmly. I said only that I understood it was hard to change treatment in this way. At the end of the session, after Clari checked that I had no long-term plans to leave the country over the next few years, we set a date for starting treatment, and I asked her to phone me a month beforehand. However, when she did call me five months later, as arranged, I was still unable to begin the treatment on the date we had set and could only begin two months later.

When Clari came in to start treatment, she appeared lost and depressed, unlike how she appeared at our first meeting. Over the previous few months, she had been very lonely, both because her therapy had ended and because her relationship with her woman friend had ended, and her friend had already formed a new relationship with another woman. She calmed down soon after treatment began, and it became apparent that the fact that treatment was taking place made her feel more held.

During the first two years of treatment that followed, she was very lonely, cut off from her former circle of women (lesbian) friends, yet resolute in her decision to establish a serious relationship with a man. Little by little, she told me that she had been repeatedly dreaming what she called "dreams of force"—horrific dreams she had had before but which were now recurring with increasing frequency. In these dreams, she was always in the familiar surroundings of her home and bedroom, when suddenly, everything would go dark, with an overpowering, sinister feeling of terror. She would usually try to do something—get up, switch on the light—without success, becoming slower, paralyzed. Then she would be gripped and overcome by a tremendous force exerting a terrible, crushing pressure on her chest and especially on her head, and she would be unable to move. She knew that there was no point in struggling; all she could do was submit and lie still until it passed so that it would spare her and not kill her and try to just continue breathing—to just survive.[3]

Despite sleeping very lightly, she could not avoid the dreams, which occurred even when she slept during the day. But gradually, over the first two years of treatment with me, the frequency of the dreams decreased, and her numerous physical pains also diminished. Clari settled into a new job and studies, and in the third year of treatment, after unsuccessfully dating several men, her relationship with her estranged husband, who over the years would phone her once a year on her birthday, was slowly and cautiously renewed. They experienced many difficulties at first; each time they quarreled, she would become frightened and threaten to end the relationship. They again encountered sexual problems, but her husband, who over the years had undergone psychotherapy, was given great, direct encouragement by his therapist to persevere in the relationship, and he showed a determination and patience that he had not had in previous years. The relationship stabilized, and they moved in together, hoping to start a family.

The zone of darkness

In moving from the description of the *events* in Clari's treatment to the treatment itself and the quality and texture of the therapeutic relationship, I enter another realm, opaque and shadowy—a zone of darkness.

From our first session in treatment, Clari spoke in a manner that was spare, restrained, vague, unclear—it is difficult for me even to find the word that might precisely describe the way she spoke. Often, I could not hear or understand what she was saying. Initially, I thought and interpreted that she found it difficult to talk to me because she had come to me for treatment against her will (and, in fact, against mine, too); but as treatment continued, there was no change. Later on, I thought that perhaps she was afraid of evolving erotic transference, or that I was afraid of it, but I quickly realized that these were rather simplistic, external interpretations. Something was strangling her capacity to communicate, but what was it?

She seemed just to need my presence there. She attended treatment regularly, never missing a session or arriving late. At the beginning of the session, she would examine me closely and then begin talking in her vague, stiff, disconnected way, her face immobile. After ten or fifteen minutes, my laborious attentiveness would gradually diminish, and I would become detached. It was not that my thoughts wandered or that I was bored. Nothing. Blank. Absent. I ceased to exist as a person who listened, thought, and responded. I would sometimes become numb and sleepy. Then, in the last ten minutes of the session, I would come out of it and become myself again, listening, relating, responding.

This pattern bore little relation to my feelings of fatigue. While at the beginning fatigue would hasten the process, later on, it made no real difference.

By the beginning of the fourth year of treatment, after the decisions and changes described earlier in Clari's life had been discussed in the treatment and actually made, and were thus less central to the therapeutic discourse, this situation became particularly acute. After the first ten to fifteen minutes of listening and responding, I would fall into a deep sleep, totally devoid of feeling. Then, in the last ten minutes, I would wake up. This was all while sitting facing her, thus I was unable to conceal it and, in fact, I did not try to.

When I first began falling asleep, Clari was very surprised that I dared close my eyes and be with her in a situation in which I was "so very unprotected and exposed." She repeatedly said that even with her woman friend, during their long relationship, over all the years of knowing each other and living together, neither ever closed her eyes in the presence of the other, not even during their intimate games and sex, because they were afraid of each other. She said that her woman friend would say that she was afraid of a streak of cold cruelty in Clari. Clari herself never dared fall soundly asleep. "As far back as I can remember, I would never sleep at night," she said.

She then began to fear that I would decide to terminate the treatment because of what was happening. Thereupon, I told her that, *indeed, something very strange was happening to me, and I could only suggest that we let things be until we could better understand what was going on* (This was what I truly thought and felt). Clari was silent for a moment and then said, "All right," in a voice I could barely hear, and she appeared very pensive and far less tense; her entire body seemed to relax. Much later, she would tell me that, throughout this entire period, up until I said this, she had been terrified that "the situation would become so unbearable that you would be unable to endure it, that you would stop breathing or stop the treatment, or that I would go mad." She was convinced that I was about to tell her that, after trying years of treatment with her, it was clear that there was no point in continuing, and that she should see another therapist. She would not be able to argue with this, as it was completely logical, but for her, it would be fatal. In her own words, "Then all is lost. We won't be saved. Death" (This, however, was only said to me much later—after shifting from psychotherapy to analysis).

But, at this stage, things continued in the same way for several months, and my direct efforts to understand my recurring sleeping, to discuss and consult, were to no avail. I examined various ideas, but felt unable to really understand or change it. I did not seem to have an inner clue for comprehending what was happening to me. My only feeling was that of a massive sinking into sleep, without emotions, without understanding, without thoughts (at the time, I didn't even ask myself or Clari what was happening to her while I was asleep). It was like something extremely dissociative, or like being under anesthesia after receiving a sleep-inducing injection. I therefore felt that I could only rely on the truth and the necessity of the treatment process, on its hidden meaning and order, and on its own reality. So I let things be and waited to see what would evolve.

This continued until one session, while still in this deep sleep, I saw a kind of schematic drawing of a bright tunnel with a small black dot moving up and down in its center. That was the first time that I saw or felt something while in this state, and I awoke with an unfamiliar sense of relief.

When Clari came to the following session, she was extremely troubled, sitting pale and silent. I waited and then remarked that she seemed troubled. She said, "No," probably because she thought I was referring to her reaction to my recurring sleeping, "Your tiredness is sometimes hard for me, but *after last time,* I thought that we are both stubborn, and when one of us weakens, the other keeps holding, and vice versa." "Yes," I said, and she gave a faint smile of relief. She fell silent again, very much within herself, and then said that she had dreamt a dream or, perhaps, hadn't dreamt at all. Perhaps it had been a kind of fantasy or a memory scene.

> *It was dark, she got up to pee, and then she saw this scene. She heard someone shouting, "No, no, no, no," a terrible cry, and she suddenly understood that it was her. Then she saw a baby, swollen from beatings, being put in a crib, a baby dressed in threadbare clothing, looking like a corpse. She saw the shadow of the person who was laying the baby down, perhaps the shadow of a woman, and she, as a little girl, was climbing up the crib's rail to see.*

This profoundly frightened her. *Who was it? Was it memory or fantasy?* It had seemed so very real—"no feeling of a dream." Was the baby her sister, who at the age of six months had become a vegetable and would lie in bed, hooked up to feeding tubes because she didn't eat? Had something happened to her? But her mother had said that even earlier, she felt there was something wrong with the baby and had taken her to all kinds of doctors. Since her sister was three years younger than she was, it seemed to fit the dream … was she herself the baby? There were the threadbare clothes, white trousers, a flannel shirt. She used to wear shabby clothes … there was an orphanage near their home, so perhaps it was something she saw there (Clari's speech was very fragmented). But, if it were her, how was she able to see it all? It was like a split within her. This frightened her greatly. She was unable to go back to sleep. She thought that this memory—the horribly battered baby—explained all the pain and the terrible somatic things she had experienced in the past: the pains in her arms and hands, the illnesses at the beginning of her marriage, the other terrible pains. Her whole body had been sick and in pain for years.

The next time she dreamt, it was again a dream of darkness, as though darkness had erupted and taken over her entire world:

> *I am outside, in the neighborhood, in a park, and suddenly it turns dark. A feeling of a power failure, and then a light failure. I can't see a thing, there's this total darkness, with no stars, no light at all. I tell myself I must go home, but it's impossible even to know which way to go, because everything is so terribly dark. There is a feeling that something dangerous is about to happen, something evil … and I woke up*

terrified, my heart pounding wildly. Darkness like the darkness before I saw the scene of the baby, like in the dream of force.

It's obvious that the darkness is an omen of bad things to come. I have to remind myself that there is life, because in some strange way, if I don't remember, if I don't hold on to reality, I'll become smaller and smaller and disappear into something like that, something dark, and empty, and suffocating. I think that the baby in the dream is me. That explains a lot of things, all the terrible somatic things. When I tell myself this, it's with a horrific feeling, of death, because it was dying, and then to live, you have to hold on to having to breathe, otherwise you'll stop. Living. Just to go on breathing. A sensation that gives me the feeling it could be reality. Not even panic, not to move, just being aware of having to breathe.

Dreams and dream-thoughts

In the period that followed, her dreams, their images, the experiences they expressed, and their sequence enabled us to get into and explore the ongoing brutal seesawing between holding and falling, hope and destruction; to recognize Clari's longing and struggle to work her way toward feeling that trust was a valid response to catastrophe. For the first time, she began dreaming different dreams, dreams of hope, of being helped, and of a helping figure. And then, in the nights that immediately followed, again, unbearable dreams, with scenes of horror and disaster. In the first different, new dream,

She goes to sleep, and in their bedroom, there is a little girl of about three, curled up and dressed only in panties. She [Clari] gets up, because she understands that if she doesn't take care of the child, no one will. She takes the child's hand and leads her into a room of her own—all is very dark, a wind is blowing and the curtains flying—and she dresses her in a nightgown. The child is happy, gets into bed, and before she falls asleep says, "I thought the whole house was going to collapse, but it's only Grandma who died."

Clari was deeply moved and fought back tears—which appeared for the first time during the treatment—when we talked about the dream. "My feeling is always kind of hazy. I have a lot of stumps," she said. "All of life is built on something that isn't there. It's like in movie cartoons—you keep going on nothing, you look down, and then you see that the ground isn't there, that you've been running on air."

Yet, each hopeful dream was immediately followed by dreams of catastrophe in which hope, change, prospects, and her sleep were attacked and shattered—although in these dreams, too, amid the shattering, now there were the beginnings of struggles for help, either in the dream or in the waking up that followed it. The night after telling me the preceding hopeful dream, Clari was thrown back into a harrowing "dream of force," in which she was in bed, and a sensation of paralysis and pressure began, particularly in her head, which was big, swollen, and heavy. She got up to turn on the light, and there was no electricity. Horrified, she tried over and over to turn on other lights, with no success, her entire body gradually becoming incapable of movement. She woke up confused and disorientated. The sensation continued for a long time; she didn't know who she was. She said to me,

> I remembered you before I remembered me. And then I said to you, to me, 'Just a second, I'm Clari, I'm 35 years old. There's Ron [her husband].' And then I told myself where I am in my life, where I work, and where I live. I almost called to tell you that something evil was about to happen, and then I realized that it wasn't real. But the sensation and the swelling in my head continued. I felt a need to eat, and I sat down and ate.

In another disastrous dream, the little girl from the previous hopeful dream was drowning, as though the good dream could not be supported for long—

> *Clari is with her husband and the little girl near a water reservoir, and the girl falls into the water. And when she falls in, she stops breathing, doesn't do a thing, curls up, and begins to sink ... the water is very deep. Clari yells to her husband to jump in and save her because the girl isn't breathing, isn't breathing. Ron begins undressing to jump into the water but has problems with his laces, and then she jumps into the water with her clothes on and begins to dive deeper underwater, but she cannot reach the little girl because the reservoir is very deep. She comes up for air and tries to dive down again, but it is clear to her that she cannot save the child. She thinks: Why doesn't Ron jump in, maybe he can reach her. It's not clear whether he jumped in or not.*

Again, the agonizing inability to be saved and to save, although there was a desperate attempt by Clari at saving.

Were the dreams heading toward a null point, a breakdown, the collapse of a new beginning?

On the threshold of analysis: between the darkness and the dread to know

Two months after the scene of the mortally battered baby, Clari asked to switch to analysis. She said she felt that she "needed to be in more treatment at this time." I agreed, but would only be able to begin analysis six months later.

Then, in the following session, a very significant one, there was a recurrence of my massive falling asleep. Clari began the session by saying, "Now that we like each other more,"—I was surprised because she had never previously used any words expressing such feelings—"I want to tell you something else." She told me that when she was a little girl, she felt she was a boy, a hyperactive boy; she would go to the bathroom and pee through a tube. She never told this to anyone, but there was something very confused in her, causing her learning difficulties and memory problems in school, in spite of her great efforts at studying. I heard her up to this point, and then I fell into a deep sleep, awaking for the last ten minutes of the session. Clari said that she was observing me "from outside," as though she were seeing the little girl sinking in the dream, as though she were seeing herself as a boy. This boy had been there since she was three years old, since nursery school. When they hit her, he was strong, so they couldn't trample her.

There was something so palpable in her words that I found myself asking, "And what was his name?"

"Johnny," she said.

I said, "You needed trust to tell me this." Apparently, I had said too much.

Clari shrank back and responded cuttingly, "Trust is needed to be here for such a long time while you sleep." She was silent; then she said, "Yes, I really never, ever told anyone about him, ever."

From this point on, she began to sleep more soundly at night, and I, during the sessions, was becoming less and less sleepy; maybe it began before, but now it was clear. The mixture of good and terrifying dreams continued, but these were dreams with a frightening content and no longer "dreams of force" in which "there is only sensation; no content." She said,

"There's no getting out of a dream of force. I'm in it; it's a horror that I can't even think. But now, when the anxiety overwhelms me, I think you and come out of it."

In addition, she would now scream in her sleep, out of the terror of the frightening dreams, screaming for help. Even when her mouth was paralyzed, and only sounds emanated, her husband would hear, wake up, and wake her. Now there was a scream, and there was someone who heard.

Then there was another change. While on the border between sleep and wakefulness, she felt herself entering her own body, and it surrounded her like a thick, flexible, safe, protective tire, whereas previously she had observed her body and kept it protected from without.

She joined her mother on a family visit to the country of her birth, and there she went to the house where she had been born, but did not dare go inside. She also did not dare to sleep during the entire journey, until her return to Israel, and treatment.

On her return, strange, unknown details of her early childhood were suddenly revealed, following a question that she asked her parents about her childhood. Her father related that when Clari was six months old, her mother suddenly developed a strange illness that tests were unable to identify, "as though life seeped out of her." He took her to the maternal grandmother's house, and he returned home and to his work. The mother was put in the cellar, in the dark, while Clari was moved to the top floor. He said that her mother would constantly ask, "Where's Clari? Where's Clari?"

What went on there? Who looked after Clari? Where was the older sister? This all remained unfathomable, unresolved, and unanswered, flooded with fantasies. The conversation caused her mother and sister great anxiety, and it was impossible to ask any further questions.

At the end of these months, prior to the shift to analysis, Clari dreamt two dreams that strongly recapitulated the motifs of falling asleep, darkness, and terror. I will conclude the clinical illustration by describing them in Clari's own words.

The first dream took place before I left for a month-long vacation, some two months before the shift to analysis; in it, there was a close connection between her being able to fall asleep, despite the dark, in face-to-face togetherness with me, and her capacity for separating afterwards.

> *It is terribly dark in here. I am lying on the couch, covered with a blanket from home, and you are sitting on a chair next to me, and then at*

> *some point you think I've fallen asleep, and you slowly get onto the couch and cover yourself. We are both lying on our sides, face-to-face, and then, in that position, I really do fall asleep, until at some point you wake me, and you're in a hurry, you have to leave, and there are all kinds of things that I dropped that you give me—car keys, my earrings, and some other things. We leave and you turn right, assuming that I'm going with you. There's a big parking lot there, but I say, "No, no, I parked on the left," and then we part.*

The second dream was just before the transition to analysis, after the session in which we finalized the two additional hours of analysis:

> *I am in my grandmother's house. The maid takes me into a room, the one that used to be mine, and when she switches on the light, the bulb burns out. It's a room that hasn't been used for a long time. She goes to get a bulb and leaves me in the dark, and I'm frightened. I ask her to take me first to the living room where everyone else is, but she already left. In the dark, I try to walk along the length of the wall, but I can't find the wall, as though there is a void all around; and yet I continue walking, with my arms out in front of me, searching for a wall, and the more I walk, the more frightening it becomes. I walk more and more slowly—these things from the dream of force, where everything begins to slow down. Eventually I can't move, I'm becoming paralyzed, with a feeling of approaching danger. By then I'm crawling and I open a door that I find. Apparently, it's the front door of the house. And then I'm even more terrified, because it's dark and I'm alone, and who knows who might come in, and I try to close the door and I can't, because I'm paralyzed. And I start to scream and scream from fear. And then someone comes in through the door, in a short skirt. She bends down and hugs me, and I see that it's my mother, and she's terribly upset, as though something very bad has happened, she's suffering a lot, and then she begins telling me that she wanted to tell the servants before she left that ... and I wake myself up because I'm so terrified, so I don't have to hear. I know that there have been times in a dream when I woke myself up, so that I wouldn't hear something.*

I thought of her desperate struggle to break through the horrific, dark void and of the moment of the encounter she described in her dream. She had forged her way out from the horror of the darkness and the void-with-no-objects in which she was left alone, and from the grip of the paralysis, and finally reached her mother. But the mother, who could have contained and mitigated the horror, was herself very upset and overwhelmed (and overwhelming) by her own distress, and Clari fears knowing her. At the threshold of the door that she now opened, on the threshold of analysis, amid the desperate helplessness, neediness, and the yearning to be helped, she fears that something unbearable has come in and will seize her through the contact with the motherly other.

Loneliness and longing, hope and dread (and the immense tension between them)—now, between the darkness and the dread to know, on the threshold of analysis...

Discussion: darkness made visible

> If the analyst can take certain steps that enable him to 'see' what the patient sees, it is reasonable to suppose that the patient has likewise 'taken steps', though not necessarily the same ones, to enable him to "see" what he sees,
>
> writes Bion (1970, p. 40)

The analyst's being- and becoming-with, or at-one-with, the patient's experiential reality—which may enable them to "see" what the patient sees—is the essence of this discussion: *"Darkness made visible."*

"Darkness made visible" was the phrase used in astrophysics to describe the first-ever picture of a black hole—a supermassive black hole at the center of galaxy M87. This marked a major transition in astrophysics: from knowing through massive influence—detecting black holes by their immense gravitational effects since their complete darkness made them invisible—to a groundbreaking collaboration among astronomers and astrophysicists that, in 2019, produced the first visual evidence of black holes in the universe.

I will address in Clari's treatment a psychic counterpart to this process of transformation—from a massive, dark, unknowable traumatic influence to a darkness made more visible and accessible, and a reaching into the most hidden, dark, and previously inaccessible depths of her psychic reality. "Darkness" and "working totally in the dark" are used both *figuratively and concretely* in this account.

Clari's treatment confronted me with abysmal not knowing and working totally in the dark, which profoundly resonated with Bion's words:

> It means that I am forced to have an emotional experience and that I have to have it in such a way that I am unable to learn from it. I have consciousness, a sense organ enabling me to perceive the psychical qualities (as Freud puts it in The Interpretation of Dreams), but I am not to be allowed to comprehend it.
>
> (1992, p. 220)

According to Winnicott's late clinical thinking (1974, 1965), this necessitates working within the unthinkable and the unexperienced until "*the thing feared has been experienced*"; or within something "more in the nature of a depersonalization or an extreme dissociation," as Winnicott refers to Scott's "regression to sleep" in Scott's presentation to the British Psycho-Analytical Society (Winnicott, January 27, 1954; in Rodman, 1987, p. 56). For Bion, this is "a nameless dread" (1962) and the "dark night of/to the soul" (words borrowed from St. John of the Cross), which is the "'dark night' to K" in analytic work (1965, p. 159). Described further in late Bion's powerful words, this is "a breakdown of dream-work-a" (1992, p. 59), "the complete dissociation" (2013, p. 68), "complete meaninglessness [when] all meaning, all source of meaning, has been annihilated" (1965, p. 101). Therefore, "The transformation in K must be replaced by the transformation in O, and K must be replaced by F [faith]" (Bion, 1970, p. 46);

> Or, as I have put it, get rid of your memory and your desire, so that you *expose yourself to the full treatment ... to being as receptive as possible. ...* the blast of an experience of this kind when you are actually there, when you are really exposed to it. It is, I can only say, 'indescribable'... It brings in *something quite different.*
>
> (1967/2013, pp. 85–86, my italics)

But darkness was also a very *concrete experience* in Clari's nightmarish psychic reality. All the gripping horror situations occur when deep darkness descends upon her familiar world, when the texture of her real, familiar, homely environment violently and abruptly collapses into something awful, unthinkable, without meaning and without mercy—something that cannot be stopped or resisted; into a complete loss of safety, confidence, protectiveness, and orientation; into near-death.

This horrifying darkness in Clari's experiential reality is intertwined with the "uncanny"—*Das Unheimliche* (Freud, 1919)—*heimlich* that becomes *unheimlich,*[4] "the class of the frightening which leads back to what is known of old and long familiar"—a lived experience (*Erlebnis*) (1919, p. 220). It is a *dark uncanny* here. Clari's dreams of horror always began in her familiar environment with the eruption and encroachment of darkness: the repeated, dreadful, overwhelming "dreams of force" occurred in the real and familiar situation of her home and bedroom; the dream/memory scene of the mortally battered baby is seen when she "got up to pee" there, in the dark; and the dream of total darkness and disorientation which immediately follows it, occurs in her familiar neighborhood.

Is this striking shift from the familiar environment to darkness, void, and repetitive horror devoid of content, an expression of an awful, extremely traumatic rupture of unthinkable anxiety, of nameless dread? Or is it also a defensive reorganization of the traumatic, horrific experiences hidden in her familiar world?

These depths of the unknown, especially the most traumatic unknown, and "being totally in the dark" figuratively and concretely, both in Clari's experiential world and in the treatment experience, necessitate going beyond epistemological exploration to the ontological analytic work of being and becoming, at-one-with the patient's innermost psychic reality—namely, the unrepressed and unrepresented realm, level **II**, in the spectrum of analytic oneness that I have proposed.

It can also be said, following Freud's thinking in "The uncanny" (1919), that I became the "double"—a human, alive, real, and present "double" in Clari's uncanniness

> by mental processes leaping from one … to another—by what we should call telepathy—so that the one possesses knowledge, feelings and experience in common with the other … there is a doubling, dividing and interchanging of the self.
>
> (p. 234)

Botella and Botella (2005) expand on the idea of the analyst's "functioning or working as a double," which goes beyond "already known" countertransference meaning and thus gives access to the patient's unrepresentable areas that would otherwise remain traumatically unknown and unreachable (pp. 82–83).

Perhaps, in order to enter and become-there within Clari's impervious, inaccessible, yet needy inner world, I had to be in an unprotected, vulnerable, even paralyzed psychic state, to match the quality of her own core vulnerability. It is an intricate match, whose essence, significance, and compatibility should be such that the analyst's/therapist's deeply interconnected presence—like a transplant or chimeric antibodies in medicine—is not identified as a foreign body by the psyche's defense system, and therefore not attacked and rejected by it, but is able to become a new, living possibility.

I would also add here Ogden's words:

> Being understood is terrifying [if] the person who understands is an other, an entirely separate person who lives outside of one's control, and at the same time knows one to the core and could, if he chose, cut one to the quick.
>
> (2016, p. 10)

But while Ogden emphasizes "a feeling of profound trust," I emphasize here the *being at one with* the patient's innermost emotional reality.

It seems to me that the massive traumatic *realness* of early breakdown and madness (Winnicott, 1974, 1965), of "psychological disaster," "primitive catastrophe," "the ruins of the psyche," and "catastrophic emotional explosion" (Bion, 1958, 1970), and "the uncanny" (Freud, 1919)—led them all toward more radical ontological forms of psychoanalytic work and transformations in oneness: in Freud—the double, "for the 'double' was originally an insurance against the destruction of the ego, an 'energetic denial of the power of death'" (Freud, 1919, p. 235); in Winnicott's and Bion's late writings, despite differences in their language, this took shape in their emphasis on the necessity of fundamental *being and experiencing* prior to understanding in the analytic work, namely, to "transformations in O" (Vermote, 2013).

To my way of thinking, this traumatic realness also shifts us from projective identification (of unbearable fear or phantasy) to what might be called *"projective realization"*[5] or *"projective embodiment" of catastrophic psychic realities that have already happened.* All this is strongly maintained in late Bion's ontological words:

> With this [O] the analyst *cannot be identified*: he must *be* it … Restating this in terms of psycho-analytic experience, the psycho-analyst can know what the patient says, does, and appears to be, but cannot know the O of which the patient is an evolution: he can only 'be' it.
>
> (1970, p. 27, italics mine and in original, respectively)

Returning to Clari's treatment

With this in mind, let us return to Clari's treatment. In Clari's psychic reality, the traumatic, terrifying early experiences were massively dissociated, their contents warded off. She was caught within a persistent, haunting scene of raw horror, with repeated, uncanny scenarios of utter darkness, loneliness, and desperation, while being in the grip of an overwhelming, inescapable anti-life force. She was crushed and stifled nearly to death, emotionally and somatically, depending for existence itself on a whim—a scene of total helplessness, of unspeakable abuse and longing, and mere physical survival. There was also the re-traumatization with which Clari came to me for treatment because of her former therapist's departure.

As the treatment evolved, Clari increasingly projected-forced these fundamental, central elements of her psychic reality into me—the coercive extreme dissociation of self-experience; the cognitive-affective paralysis with the gap in continuity of experience (Lichtenberg et al., 1992); the absence. Now, the experience of being inside a massive dissociative, blank process was occurring in *me—a vicarious self-state dissociation,* thus detaching and distancing it from her while she observed from without. But when I let it affect me, allowing it to be and become me, without understanding it but also without dread, carrying in me the experience of having been repeatedly dissociated and absent—yet staying there, in the treatment, surviving, trying to hold and think the experience—it gradually became a therapeutic experience. The dissociation very slowly became a new kind of dissociation—*an attenuated, deferred dissociation*, because the dissociation in me—or, more precisely, in the interconnected entity of her-and-me—was no longer the extremely lonely, unmediated, life-defending dissociative self-experience of her, but a dissociative experience that was held differently within me, and within a human process—a massive yet sustained and tolerable one.

I quoted earlier Bion's words

> If the analyst can take certain steps that enable him to 'see' what the patient sees, it is reasonable to suppose that the patient has likewise 'taken steps', though not necessarily the same ones, to enable him to 'see' what he sees.
>
> (1970, p. 40)

And indeed, after months of my unchanging recurring sleep in Clari's treatment,

> one session, while still in this deep sleep, I saw a kind of schematic drawing of a bright tunnel with a small black dot moving up and down in its center. This was the first time that I saw or felt something while in this state, and I awoke with an unfamiliar sense of relief.

And although I was unable to put it into words for me or for her, Clarie came to the next session and told me the horrible dream/memory scene of the mortally battered baby.

Thus, the externalization of the dissociation within and through me, and being within psyche-to-psyche connectedness, enabled Clari to dare approach, observe, and experience the dread of her inner self-other experiences. She could begin to dream, think, imagine, to risk exploring the traumatic contents of her massive uncanniness, which, until then, had been unknowable, unthinkable, extremely dissociated, and inaccessible, threatening her with desperation, collapse, madness, and dying. Fact-finding became self-finding. In this way, we went through and beyond the complete dissociation.

Finally, still along this line of deep patient-analyst interconnectedness, but looking at my "sleep" from a very different perspective—my sleep during Clari's treatment could be regarded as a regression in the countertransference to a "good sleep" (suggested by Bollas, 1997, personal communication). When I actualized the capacity to fall asleep for Clari, she, too, was able to let herself fall soundly asleep (as in the dream of her falling asleep, in spite of the dark, in face-to-face togetherness with me). She could hold the hand of the terrified, lost little girl within herself and put her to bed, as in the first good dream that she dreamt, and begin to actualize "dream-space" (Khan, 1972) and inner space for remembering, which she was robbed of by her traumatic childhood. This is a "good sleep" that is created with and through another person. This point resonates with Ferenczi's (1932) early words: "A sleeping person is defenseless: When one is asleep, one relies on the safety of the house and the environment, otherwise one could not fall asleep" (p. 45).

> Wherever you find yourself with a patient, you have to go. We wish things could be otherwise, could be easier, but we have little choice when light shines through the ruins of injury. I think that is a very Kabbalistic model.
>
> (Eigen, 2005, p. 41)

I think that is also the very essence of the ontological-experiential model of "presencing," withnessing and at-one-ment. Perhaps only a withnessing-enough process could stand a chance.

So perhaps, at the end of all the explanations and beyond all explanations, I would dare to say that in this treatment, without knowing it at the time, amid the depths of not understanding and not knowing, there came into being an *"act of faith"* (Bion, 1970) and "area of faith" (Eigen, 1981)—out of my fundamental, profound belief and trust in the psychoanalytic process, in the deep connectedness of patient-and-analyst, in myself as an analyst; and not less important—out of Clari's persistence in treatment which grew into her great determination to intensify it, despite the dread that was strongly expressed in her dream just prior to the transition to analysis, as she opened the door to the unknown. It was an "act of faith" that came into being within the evolving oneness of me-and-Clari, Clari-and-me.

Afterword

In this account, I have restricted myself to what I experienced, came to understand, and did not understand about my "sleeping"—during the course of Clari's psychotherapy and shortly afterwards, at the beginning of the analysis. I chose not to use material from later in the analysis because I wanted to convey the quality of the experience for me at the time—its grip, its experiential vicissitudes, its unknowns and unfoldings. Yet, I would like to add that during the analysis, I no longer experienced "sleeping." It seems that this was a phase in the treatment that Clari and I had already lived through. *T(w)ogether.*

Notes

1 In modern physics, different paradigms of classical physics and quantum mechanics co-exist. Whereas classical physics (and classical psychoanalysis) are based on assumptions of linear causality, determinism, and a sharp separation between observer and observed, quantum physics introduced into scientific thinking essential principles of uncertainty and inseparability of observer and observed, the crucial formative effect of the process of observation, and the fundamental organization of unbroken wholeness that underlies our perceived world of separateness at the fundamental particle level. Thus, as classical physics and quantum mechanics coexist in modern physics, classical psychoanalysis and a quantum psychoanalytic perspective may also coexist within psychoanalysis (Eshel, 2017, 2019a).

2 "Be at one with" (Bion, 1967, 1970); "become 'at-one' with the patient's experience" (F. Bion, 1995, pp. 96, 107); "Being-at-one-with" (Winnicott, 1971, p. 94).

3 Regarding this dream, I encountered an article in *The New York Times* that described phenomena such as a sensed presence, terror, strong immobility, a crushing pressure, and struggle for breath as the mysterious "sleep paralysis" (Kristof, 1999).
4 When I asked a native German speaker to explain the word *unheimlich*, she said, "It is a child in darkness, a lurking danger."
5 Also Wassermann, 2021, but in a somewhat different sense.

References

Abram, J. (2013). Introduction & Notes for the Vienna Congress 1971: A consideration of Winnicott's theory of aggression and an interpretation of the clinical implication (2012). In J. Abram (ed.), *Donald Winnicott Today,* 2013 (pp. 1–25; pp. 302–330). London/New York: Routledge/The New Library of Psychoanalysis.
Bergstein, A. (2014). Beyond the spectrum: Fear of breakdown, catastrophic change and the unrepressed unconscious. *Rivista Di Psicoanalisi*, 60: 847–868.
Bion, F. (1995). The days of our years. In C. Mawson (ed.), *The Complete Works of W. R. Bion, Vol. XV* (pp. 91–111). London: Karnac, 2014.
Bion, W. R. (1958). On arrogance. In *Second Thoughts* (pp. 86–92). London: Maresfield Library/Karnac, 1967.
Bion, W.R. (1959). Attacks on linking. In *Second Thoughts* (pp. 93–109). London: Maresfield Library/Karnac, 1967.
Bion, W. R. (1962). *Learning from Experience*. London: Maresfield Library/Karnac.
Bion, W. R. (1965). *Transformations*. London: Maresfield Library/Karnac.
Bion, W. R. (1967). Notes on memory and desire. *The Psychoanalytic Forum*, 2: 272–273.
Bion, W. R. (1970). *Attention and Interpretation*. London: Maresfield Library/Karnac.
Bion, W. R. (1992). *Cogitations*. London: Karnac.
Bion, W. R. (2005). *The Italian Seminars*. London and New York: Karnac.
Bion, W. R. (2013). *Los Angeles Seminars and Supervisions*. Eds. J. Aguayo & B. Malin. London: Karnac.
Bohm, D. (1980). *Wholeness and the Implicate Order*. London: Routledge/Kegan Paul.
Bollas, C. (1997). Personal communication.
Botella, C. & Botella, S. (2005). *The Work of Psychic Figurability: Mental States without Representation.* Hove and New York: Brunner-Routledge/The New Library of Psychoanalysis.
Braga, J. C. (2021). *Pathways to at-one-ment: Withnessing, Receptivity and Reverie*. IPA Congress, June, 2021.
Braga, J. C. (2022). A different perspective on at-one-ment: Discussion of Ofra Eshel's "Transformations on oneness." São Paulo´s Brazilian Psychoanalytic Society, April, 2022.

Bromberg, P.M. (2006). *Awakening the Dreamer: Clinical Journeys*. Mahwah, N.J.: Analytic Press.
Bromberg, P.M. (2011). *The Shadow of the Tsunami and the Growth of the Relational Mind*. New York: Routledge.
de M'Uzan, M. (2006). Invitation to frequent the shadows. *European Psychoanalytical Federation Bulletin, 60*, 14–28.
Eigen, M. (1981). The area of faith in Winnicott, Lacan, and Bion. *International Journal of Psychoanalysis*, 62: 413–433.
Eigen, M. (2005). Interview with Micha Odenheimer. *Another Country (Eretz Acheret)*, 26: 36–42.
Eshel, O. (2001). Whose sleep is it, anyway? Or "Night Moves". *International Journal of Psychoanalysis*, 82: 545–562.
Eshel, O. (2004). Let it be and become me: Notes on containing, identification, and the possibility of being. *Contemporary Psychoanalysis*, 40: 323–351.
Eshel, O. (2017). From extension to revolutionary change in clinical psychoanalysis: The radical influence of Bion and Winnicott. *Psychoanalytic Quarterly*, 86(4): 753–794.
Eshel, O. (2019a). *The Emergence of Analytic Oneness: Into the Heart of Psychoanalysis*. London and New York: Routledge.
Eshel, O. (2019b). The vanished last scream: Winnicott and Bion. *Psychoanalytic Quarterly*, 88(1), 111–140.
Eshel, O. (2021). Pathways to At-one-ment – Let it Be and Become Me: Transformations in Oneness. Presentation at the International Psychoanalytic Association Congress, Vancouver, Canada, November.
Eshel, O. (2023). When deadness breaks in: Surviving, 'being-with' and a moment of 'at-one-ment' in analytic work within deadness and emptiness. *Modern Psychoanalysis*, 47: 145–171.
Eshel, O. (2025a). Being totally in the dark: On working analytically within the depths of the great unknown of psychic catastrophe. In D. Power & D. Power (eds.), *The somato-psychic realm: Analytic receptivity and resonance* (pp. 82–103). London and New York: Routledge.
Eshel, O. (2025b). "Must have a mathematics of at-one-ment, not identification": Theoretical reflections and three clinical examples. Presentation at the 13th Bion International conference, New York, June.
Eshel, O. (2026). "Must have a mathematics of at-one-ment, not identification": The Breakthrough of Late Bion. Presentation at the Sichuan Heguang Institute, China, January.
Eshel, O. & Zeligman, Z. (2017). *Was It or Was It Not? When Shadows of Sexual Abuse Emerge in Psychoanalytic Treatment*. Jerusalem: Carmel.
Ferenczi, S. (1932). 24 February 1932: Trauma in an unconscious state. In J. Dupont (ed.), M. Balint & N. Z. Jackson (trans.), *The Clinical Diary of Sandor Ferenczi* (pp. 45–32). Cambridge, MA and London: Harvard Univ. Press, 1988.

Ferro, A. (2021). Foreword. In H. B. Levine (ed.), *The Post-Bionian Field Theory of Antonio Ferro: Theoretical Analysis and Clinical Applications* (pp. x–xiii). London and New York: Routledge.
Freud, S. (1900). The interpretation of dreams (Part 2). *SE*, 5: 339–627.
Freud, S. (1915). The unconscious. *SE*, 14: 161–215.
Freud, S. (1919). The 'uncanny'. *SE*, 17: 217–253.
Freud, S. (1923). The ego and the id. *SE*, 19: 31–66.
Green, A. (1973) On negative capability – A critical review of W.R. Bion's "Attention and Interpretation." *International Journal of Psychoanalysis,* 54:115–119.
Khan, M. M. (1972). The use and abuse of dream in psychic experience. In *The Privacy of the Self* (pp. 306–315). London: Hogarth, 1974.
Kohut, H. (1984). *How Does Analysis Cure?* A. Goldberg & P. Stepansky (eds.). Chicago: University of Chicago Press.
Kristof, N. D. (1999). Alien abduction? Science calls it sleep paralysis. *The New York Times*, 7 July 1999.
Levine, H. B. (2022). *Affect, Representation and Language: Between the Silence and the Cry.* London and New York: Routledge.
Levine, H., Reed, G. S. & Scarfone, D. (eds.) (2013). *Unrepresented States and the Construction of Meaning: Clinical and Theoretical Contribution.* London: Karnac.
Lichtenberg, J. D., Lachmann, F. M. & Fosshage, J. L. (1992). *Self and Motivational Systems: Toward a Theory of Psychoanalytic Technique.* Hillsdale, NJ and London: Analytic Press.
Meltzer, D. (1967). The Psychoanalytic Process. London: Karnac.
Ogden, T. H. (2001). Reading Winnicott. In *Conversations at the Frontier of Dreaming* (pp. 203–235). London & New York: Karnac.
Ogden, T. H. (2016). *Reclaiming Unlived Life.* London and New York: Routledge.
Ogden, T. H. (2019). Ontological psychoanalysis or "what do ou want to be when you grow up?" *Psychoanalytic Quarterly*, 88(4): 661–684.
Rodman, R. F. (ed.) (1987). *The Spontaneous Gesture: Selected Letters of D.W. Winnicott* (pp. 89–93). Harvard University Press.
Searles, H. F. (1965) *Collected Papers on Schizophrenia and Related Subjects.* London: Maresfield.
Stern, D. B. (2015). *Relational Freedom: Emergent Properties of the Interpersonal Field.* London and New York: Routledge.
Stern, D. B. (2019). *The Infinity of the Unsaid.* London and New York: Routledge.
Vermote, R. (2013). *The undifferentiated zone of psychic functioning: An integrative approach and clinical implications.* Presentation at the European Psychoanalytical Federation (EPF) Conference, Basel, March 24. See also: Vermote, R. (2013). The undifferentiated zone of psychic functioning. *European Psychoanalytical Federation, Psychoanalysis in Europe Bulletin*, 67: 16–27.
Winnicott, D. W. (1945). Primitive emotional development. In *Through Paediatrics to Psychoanalysis* (pp. 145–156). London: Karnac Books and the Institute of Psycho-Analysis, 1992.

Winnicott, D. W. (1963). Communicating and not communicating leading to a study of certain opposites. In *The Maturational Processes and the Facilitating Environment* (pp. 179–192). London: Hogarth Press, 1979.
Winnicott, D. W. (1965). The psychology of madness: A contribution from psychoanalysis. In C. Winnicott R. Shepherd & M. Davis (eds.), *Psycho-analytic Explorations* (pp. 119–129). London: Karnac Books, 1989.
Winnicott, D. W. (1971). *Playing and Reality*. Harmondsworth: Penguin.
Winnicott, D. W. (1974). Fear of breakdown. *International Review of Psycho-Analysis*, 1: 103–107.

Chapter 2

Into the wilderness with Ofra Eshel and her patient Clari[1]

Charles Levin

Introduction

Ofra Eshel speaks and writes with a passion that is rare in the world of psychoanalysis, and she puts her passion to work in ways that are unusual in the profession. I believe that the implications of her work are consequential and cannot be identified clearly within the conventions of psychoanalytic discourse. The intensity and depth of her thinking belong to psychoanalysis, but they stretch the field beyond its customary limits. This has something to do with the quality of her "persona." She speaks with the voice of a skilled clinician and creative theoretician, but her passion brims over into another register of communication from which the psychoanalytic profession generally shies away. I shall explore several aspects of this phenomenon. I shall try to describe in detail how her work undermines standard accounts of what it means to 'connect' with an analytic patient. In order to illustrate this point, I will take the liberty, in the first part of this paper, of reframing her avowed debts to Winnicott and especially Bion. In the second part, I will explore some implications of her remarkable relationship with Clari.

Part 1. Bion, plus or minus?

It bears repeating that Ofra Eshel is an exceptional writer. Her book, *The Emergence of Analytic Oneness: Into the Heart of Psychoanalysis* (2019), needs to be read in its entirety. It is more than a useful compendium of her clinical insight over the years; it is also a searing commentary on the state of human civilization at this major junction in the troubled history of our species on this planet. In that sense, her book is an important contribution to contemporary social thought, in the tradition of Freud and the late Bion. As I think Eshel makes clear in her references to the literary

DOI: 10.4324/9781003674078-4

and cultural traditions of our Abrahamic civilization, we are at the brink of what Bion called the "Dawn of Oblivion" (Bion, 1991). We can hear the screams of her patients, and to my ear, they are also the screams of human history—verging on what she describes as "the last cry before hope was abandoned" (2019, p. 18). Reading her reminds me of a famous passage in Walter Benjamin's *Theses on the Philosophy of History*, in which he interpreted Paul Klee's water color, *Angelus Novus*, as the suffering "angel of history." When Benjamin wrote this, he knew the Shoah was coming. In his comments on Klee's image (which visually resembles the Greek letter *psi* [Ψ]), Benjamin (1969) saw the angel of history frozen in the air, with his back turned to the future, his wings spread out and pinned open by the onrushing gale of human catastrophe.

Eshel's work embraces one of the central paradoxes of the psychoanalytic tradition. Psychoanalysis has always been poised on the cusp of a practical and moral dilemma: are we treating the suffering of the individual, or are we engaged in what is essentially a critique of the human condition? I believe that the spirit of psychoanalysis necessarily includes both of these 'knowledge interests'[2] (Habermas, 1972), but there seems to be no way to totalize psychoanalytic thought by fully integrating the two perspectives theoretically. Lewis Kirschner (2011) in his study *Between Winnicott and Lacan* has envisaged "the possibility of a psychoanalytic treatment that can move between two seemingly incompatible theories of the origins and structure of the human psyche" (2011, p. ix). Eshel's thinking moves in this dialectical way, unfolding in complex tension with the ultimately irreconcilable polarities of the psychoanalytic spectrum of thought—the project of social and intellectual *critique* of civilization on the one hand, which Freud favored temperamentally, even in his early clinical theory of neurosis; and on the other what might be called the *pastoral or therapeutic* functions of psychoanalysis. Eshel situates herself squarely on the therapeutic side of this spectrum. At the same time, she has developed a wider orientation to human suffering.

Freud believed at first that these two competing knowledge interests—critical thinking versus the pastoral address to suffering—were really one and the same thing, at least in the sense that truth (or the search thereof) would itself be the primary agent of cure. This was, of course, an Enlightenment article of faith, encapsulated in Kant's slogan, *sapere aude*! (dare to know), which in psychoanalytic terms translates naturally into the classical formula of making the unconscious conscious by means of interpretation. In this sense, Freud seemed to pitch the 'talking cure' as a compassionate administering of critical reason.[3] But of course, he had no such delusions. From the very beginning, as he developed his first ideas about infantile sexuality, he understood that from the perspective of social reality, psychoanalysis was bound to be perceived as dangerous and risky.[4]

The double constitution of psychoanalysis as both critical reason and therapeutic reason can be framed in terms of the conceptual distinction Kirschner (2011, pp. ix–xii) proposed between the concept of the subject and the concept of the self. From this perspective, we can see the critical aim of psychoanalysis as concerned primarily with developing a detailed investigation of the subject position within the social order to which the individual analysand is subjected: in that sense, psychoanalysis poses a critical challenge to society, as in Freud's original understanding of sexuality. On the other hand, we can see the therapeutic or 'pastoral' aim of psychoanalysis as concerned primarily with the welfare of a particular *self*—in the sense of the personal 'being' of one who may or may not be psychically 'alive' in the Winnicottian sense. Eshel's work suggests that the pastoral treatment of the 'self' can also have a powerful critical edge. Her psychoanalytic outlook combines the therapeutic interest in treating the individual patient as a damaged 'self' with a wider perspective on the individual as an exemplar of human suffering. If the psychoanalytic therapy of the self is to reach its fullest potential, it must necessarily put into play an 'ontological hazard'—not only for the patient, but for the analyst as well. A brief digression on the relation of her work to Winnicott and Bion will serve to highlight Eshel's originality in this regard.

Although her intuitive sense of the need for what she calls 'presencing' preceded her discovery of Winnicott and Bion (Eshel, 2019, p. 27), Eshel has pointedly acknowledged her debt to these authors and her gratitude to them (see especially Eshel, 2019, pp. 237–271). I shall be arguing that the implications of her own clinical work go well *beyond* what they envisaged, especially with regard to the question of how *the analyst connects with the patient* and what she describes as "the essential role of the analyst's presence" (2019, p. 27). This, I believe, is especially the case for Bion. There are strong theoretical and attitudinal reasons to understand her work as being more fundamentally aligned with Winnicott's contributions than those of Bion. Winnicott was intensely humanistic in his outlook and deeply concerned with the welfare of individual human casualties of environmental failure. In this sense, he was a 'pastoral or therapeutic' analyst through and through and thus, at least in this regard, close in spirit to Eshel's way of working.

In terms of the internal tension between the critical versus therapeutic/pastoral aims of psychoanalysis, Bion may appear to fall somewhere in the middle of the spectrum, given his avid interest in epistemology and philosophy on the one hand and his evident devotion to clinical psychoanalysis on the other. There are many who, in different ways, have understood his work as a beautiful synthesis of psychoanalysis and philosophy (most recently, Civitarese, 2025). Be that as it may, it is difficult to ignore the textual evidence of a gap—or even a contradiction—between Bion's formal theories of psychoanalysis and the way he wrote and spoke about his own clinical work.[5] He presented himself consistently as aloof toward patients, somewhat sardonic, and surprisingly argumentative. A tendency to get unnecessarily tangled up in practical criticism of the patient's misguided thinking emerges clearly in his Brazilian consultations.[6] Many of his own case vignettes and supervisory consultations were actually comic stories at the expense of the patient, as in his Rabelaisian account of a stutterer on his couch (CW 10, pp. 15–21). We can recognize in these tendencies the need to insulate oneself in what Bion called "The Analyst's Odyssey" (*Cogitations*, CW 11, see esp. pp. 211–213).

Bion's case narratives frequently address a clinical process that he describes as empty and lifeless, in which he sits back in bemused fashion as things go steadily from bad to worse. For some reason, he would get too involved with the members of the patient's family and social circle; he was nearly always angry at the patient; and he was generally sarcastic about what the patient would bring to the sessions. In one disastrous example (CW 7, pp. 126–134), after a frustrating year at the rate of five sessions a week, Bion toys with the idea of the patient committing suicide: "I was able to draw the patient's attention to the feeling that if he … became a famous patient, then at last he would feel that it was worth killing himself" (p. 131). Bion remained in this state of resentful detachment until finally the patient did commit suicide. Someone in the Rio de Janeiro audience commented to Bion, apparently in admiration, that "In the case you cited, the analyst's role seems to help the patient to die, since he cannot help him to live" (CW 7, p. 134). Bion's reply was non-committal: "The analyst's function is to analyze. It is like being a mirror being held up to the patient…" (CW 7, p. 134).

Bion was certainly trying to help his patients, but there are few grounds for assuming that he was a pioneer in the advancement of analytic technique; in spite of all his alphanumerical coruscations, in clinical technical terms he never got much beyond the classical interpretation-centered model that we have inherited from Freud. In his writings about analytic method, Bion was less interested in therapeutic problems than in a certain *idea* of psychoanalysis, and therefore in its idealized theory, whether scientific-deductive or mytho-poetic. Throughout his writings, from the early schizophrenia papers onward, one can sense Bion's wariness and distrust of actual psychoanalytic patients.

Nonetheless, certain very substantial Bionian ideas have found their way into Eshel's work for important reasons. As noted earlier, Eshel's psychoanalytic outlook combines the therapeutic interest in treating the individual patient as a damaged 'self' with a wider perspective on the individual as an exemplar of human suffering. Eshel's ardent spiritual overview of the human condition is always shimmering in the background of her work. This is where I think Bion's influence best fits into her way of thinking—in contradistinction to the more clinically challenging question of how to actually *reach* the patient.

In her introduction to the case of Clari, Eshel (2019, p. 66) tells us that

> over the years, I have come to think of extreme experiences in the clinical situation as a challenge to one's technique and complacent knowing. They evoke search and struggle, ingenuity and creative moves, at times leading us to extend and even go beyond, the boundaries of our understanding and knowledge. They are an *internal Rubicon that we have to cross*.
>
> (emphasis added)

In my understanding of Bion, he never seems to have imagined crossing an "internal Rubicon" in a "search and struggle" to reach the patient in the sense Eshel describes. He may indeed have been an "ontological" analyst (Ogden, 2019); and we can see how this understanding of his work might be supported by his later language, such as 'ultimate reality,' 'Godhead,' 'being in O,' 'becoming O,' 'at-one-ment,' and so on. Eshel has come to adopt many of these terms in her effort to situate what she does within a familiar theoretical framework. But as Bion's case presentations in the Los Angeles and Buenos Aires seminars make clear, he was not interested in crossing any internal Rubicon; he expected his patients to conform to his theoretical assumptions about a proper psychoanalytic process. If they went along with him but didn't get much better, there was always the explanation that perhaps they were psychotic. If they failed to comply, he would simply pull rank on them. Bion did recognize the need to adapt to certain patients, but he viewed this as a kind of annoying imposition:

> It's no good arguing … sooner or later the patients' revolt will take the form of demanding that people exist who can deal with their trouble … You really have to be the kind of personality who will do the job while this kind of business is going on.
>
> (Aguayo & Malin, 2013, p. 86)

He would scold, and he would even engage in intellectual mind-games, which bordered on gaslighting the patient, even to the point of imposing what he called "discipline" (Aguayo et al., 2018, pp. 69–70ff; pp. 73–74).[7]

We can explain these anomalous features of Bion's clinical discourse in various ways, but one thing is clear: Dr. Eshel's psychoanalytic style, including her account of her work with Clari, offers a compelling contrast. She is a remarkably creative clinician whose explorations of the clinical unknown are an inspiration to many, myself included. Her narrative of the extraordinary clinical journey she took with Clari is striking for its vivid illustration (typical of Eshel's case studies) of the circuitous paths taken by the analytic couple together through an obstacle course of despair, alienation, and maddening separateness, in syncopation with an enigmatic form of unspoken intimacy and somato-psychic intermingling that takes root and blossoms even when at points they seem more distant from each other than ever. Citing Harold Searles, Eshel invites us to consider what may happen when

> both patient and therapist become immersed in and swept forward by the current, the process, of treatment… [N]ot only the patient but the therapist also is in the grip of the therapeutic process … which … is far too powerful for either the patient or the therapist [to control].
>
> (Eshel, 2019, p. 68)

These important words convey a clinical spirit very different from Bion's. With regard to the current and flow of the analytic process, it is important to recognize that the best Bion could do was to talk abstractly about the "evolution of O," in which the analyst's O might *intersect* with the patient's at some point along their separate tracks (1970, p. 118; CW 6, p. 321). Bion had no way of describing in experiential terms what he meant by "at-one-ment" or being at-one with the patient. All he could say was that the analyst has to "become infinite" (1970, p. 46; CW 6, p. 259). Bion did not think of the psychoanalytic process as embracing both participants simultaneously, sweeping them away "*two*gether" into the wilderness of the psychic unknown, as Dr. Eshel so beautifully describes.

Eshel comes much closer than Bion to giving us a sense of what the phrase "at one" might signify. She describes the giving over of herself to the patient ("suspending … her own subjective reality") through a kind of emptying out of herself. The process she describes is reminiscent in some ways of the theological concept of *kenosis*, through which Christ is thought to have opened himself to humanity by evacuating his own divinity. With great passion, citing Michael Eigen, she describes

> the analyst's difficult, sometimes exceedingly difficult, struggle to give himself/herself over—with all one's heart, soul, might … to being there within the troubled emotional experience of the patient's world—staying open and attuned, sensing, hearing, and feeling the 'voice' of the patient's trauma or breakdown that cries out.
>
> (Eshel, 2019, pp. 12–13)

Eshel's emphasis on suspending her own subjective reality (p. 38) and giving herself over to the patient's world, or what I would call "narcissistic surrender to the patient," is reminiscent of de M'Uzan's (1976) "paradoxical transference." De M'Uzan described intricate dynamics in which the analyst finds themself "in a state of alert towards the object, and his own sense of identity [has] changed … as if he had evacuated what was most personal in him, while, at the same time, his psychic apparatus had become particularly permeable…" (1976, p. 19).

Eshel's formulations of her clinical work—for example, her telling phrase "crossing the internal Rubicon"—suggest to me the idea that as psychoanalysts we are not so much exploring the 'depths' of the mind, in the classical sense, as the potentials of psychoanalytic space itself. This is a broad question that lies at the heart of current psychoanalytic debate. It is not likely to be settled here, of course. I will simply underline the obvious—that the central issue in Eshel's work is the challenge of how to connect with a patient who is, for all practical purposes, unreachable in psychoanalytic or any other terms. I am referring, of course, to that aspect in the shaping of our psychic lives that may be literally unspeakable, and, for some people, unliveable. As Eshel shows so beautifully with her concepts of 'presencing' and 'withnessing' that may deepen into 'at-onement,' the psychoanalytic relationship has the potential to provide a secure expressive space in which these inarticulate and obscure layers and sources of human suffering can be, for lack of a better word, 'enacted' and thus explored within the framework of a lived experience that is shared. This possibility depends upon the analyst's receptivity to the unthinkable dimensions of their own being, which may be reverberating in response to the patient and the psychic environment being generated through their relationship. We sometimes call this "the field." Dr. Eshel's perspective on this question suggests a way of going even further; it may usefully be integrated with current neuroscientific and phenomenological conceptions of the 'embodied mind,' in which cognition itself is understood as a form of body-environment enaction (Varela et al., 2016). I believe this approach fits well with the kind of post-Winnicottian work that Dr. Eshel is doing. One of Winnicott's (1949) fundamental insights was that 'mind,' in the traditional dualistic or Cartesian sense, involves only a small and fundamentally dissociated aspect of what he called the psyche-soma.

In considering these possibilities, however, we need to keep in mind some of the differences between Winnicott writing in the mid-twentieth century, under the shadow of Klein and in the wake of Freud's death, and Eshel writing now. Winnicott's concepts of holding and 'regression to dependence' provide an important bridge to her concepts of 'presencing' and 'withnessing.' However, the latter should not be reduced to Winnicott's theory of maternal holding—nor to Bion's somewhat more paternalistic theory of containment. Eshel has reimagined the analytic relationship in a configuration that is less redolent of the standard object-relations imagery of a prepotent begetter, the idealized good object who must be worshipped (Meltzer, 1981, p. 179); she speaks more in the horizontal register, evoking a form of uncanny communication between 'fellow beings,' relying less than most of us on the traditional vertical parental model of responsible control and boundary-setting.

Eshel's practical understanding of the dimensions of psychic life is consistent with the neurological-phenomenological model of the "embodied mind" that has been developing since the ground-breaking work of Varela et al. (2016). Current neurological research can be linked to basic aspects of Freudian thought (see, for example, Solms, 2023), but with clinical implications that vary significantly from the classical model of treatment. Current understandings of the brain as a "prediction machine" (Carhart-Harris & Friston, 2010; Clark, 2023), a biological regulatory system that is engaged in an ongoing process of "active inference," align fairly well with Freud's standard metapsychology, but they do not support a view of the psyche as a closed system that is ontologically isolated from "external reality." The phenomenological interpretation of current neuroscientific and neonatological research suggests that psychic life is an emergent property of the body in ongoing interaction and negotiation with others and with the physical and cultural environment.

The concept of the embodied mind aims to overcome our deeply entrenched dualistic assumptions but also the overly localized counter-conception of mind as brain. It proposes that human bodies are interdependent with the environment, at all levels of intelligence, as self-organizing systems. All cognition is enactive, and certain basic kinds of mental functioning require the activation of the whole body-environment complex. I think it is reasonable to expect that the same principles would apply in our thinking psychoanalytically about the psyche-soma (in Winnicott's sense of the term). From this perspective, we might describe the specific psychoanalytic dimension as 'the inter-corporeal' or 'inter-embodied' unconscious. It is obviously not possible to provide a precise map of such a domain, but we can sense its wide experiential parameters in Dr. Eshel's clinical examples. Thus, we can say that in psychoanalysis the *psyche* is embodied, embedded, extended, and enactive in ecological[8] and cultural space and time (see Varela et al., esp. Chapter 8; also Gallagher, 2005). Eshel's psychoanalytic way of working with her patients fits naturally into this integrative model of the mind-world problem.[9]

Part 2. Into the wilderness with Clari

Crossing the internal Rubicon

In discussing the case of Clari, I do not wish to enter into a supervisory discussion of the material, as if in the service of some idealized fantasy of what psychoanalysts should do. I shall suggest a few ideas, but my starting point is rather the singularity of Eshel's relationship with Clari, and the utter eccentricity of the process of treatment that unfolded, during which for a considerable time, Eshel was swept along in the current of the analytic process in an unconventional, but highly relevant way, by falling into a deep and featureless sleep near the beginning of each session, only to resurface, so to speak, ten minutes before the end.

I use the word '*singularity*' here because, if we just try to think about what Eshel is showing us in this case, independently of her Bionian theoretical language, what we discover is that when it comes to the clinical bottom line, psychoanalysis really has no specific form, no standard or core technique. Yes, to be sure, we enjoy all the benefit and wisdom of our analytic training, learning, and experience. But at the primordial level where Eshel dares to go, there is in the final analysis only this unique and eccentric contingency, the singularity, which her work with Clari so beautifully exemplifies. This is something that cannot be predicted, planned, or codified. It is not something that we can prepare ourselves for epistemologically, as Bion tried to persuade us we can do. The sum and the sense of it, beyond the idea of 'being in O,' is that with this particular patient, at this particular time, Eshel needed to fall asleep in the sessions. We have no credible theory of this, and in principle we cannot expect to have one, because it is a contingent phenomenon with no known etiology. As Eshel says, if we are going to go into the wilderness with our patients, as some of them desperately need us to do, we have to "cross the internal Rubicon."

She writes:

> My only feeling was that of a massive sinking into sleep, without emotions, without understanding, without thoughts ... It was like something extremely dissociative, or like being under anaesthesia after receiving a sleep-inducing injection. I therefore felt that I could only rely on the truth and the necessity of the treatment process, on its hidden meaning and order, and on its reality. So I let things be and waited to see what would evolve.

If we think carefully about the way Dr. Eshel uses Winnicott and Bion, we realize that when she cites them as a precedent for her analytic approach, it is not so much in terms of any theory of mind or technique, but rather in this emphasis on the singularity of the patient—what Hannah Arendt (1958, p. 9) called '*natality*.'[10] For me (and I think Eshel too), this means not only that every patient is an exception to the rule in psychoanalysis, but also that every analyst, as Bion (1980, p. 27) sometimes said, will have to deal with this exception in their own way.

Eshel's work with Clari illustrates the clinical action of unpremeditated surrender; she describes the moment of criticality where, with some patients, the state of evenly suspended attention (whether we define it as reverie, or as the analyst's free association), simply breaks down. At this point, the analyst has no recourse to a prescribed analytic state of mind or technique. For all intents and purposes, the analyst has ceased to function as a container—or for that matter, even as the one who 'holds.' What Dr. Eshel does in this situation is very different in certain key respects from what Bion or Winnicott describe. With Clari, and her other more challenging patients, she stays in steadfast *receptivity* beyond the point at which one is able to receive information about the patient's state of being by ordinary psychoanalytic methods. Of course, all of this depends upon the analyst's confidence in their own intuition, their trust in going where they feel themselves being taken. It is a risky process. Eshel once referred to it as the "venture zone" (2004). At this point of criticality, only in the most conventional sense of being the paid clinician does Eshel retain any semblance of 'control' over her own mental processes. Otherwise, theoretically and practically, she is pretty much in the wilderness with Clari.

As I have already mentioned, I think of Eshel's approach to the analysand as a kind of therapeutically motivated surrender—essentially a narcissistic one (cf. M'Uzan, 1976, 1978). The main point is that when facing the "internal Rubicon" she describes, the analyst has no recourse to any technical precept. One cannot just say: "Oh dear, I'd better start becoming O"—or: "I should be eschewing more memory and desire." In situations like these, we are left with little else than an attitude of commitment—a willingness to keep on going, in spite of everything. This is a sort of personal defiance in the face of unimaginable pain and suffering. As Samuel Beckett (1965, p. 444) famously said, "I can't go on, I'll go on."

What Eshel is implicitly teaching is that the analyst must be able to accept the collapse of the prescribed analytic function, the disruption of the trained capacity to receive, digest and think. The analyst must give up their ego-syntonic professional identifications and "cross the internal Rubicon." It is in this *unwilled* acceptance of analytic incapacity that Bion's rhetoric of Faith begins to make sense. What Eshel describes is a situation in which the only way forward is a 'pastoral or therapeutic' surrender to total devastation in the field, in which the analyst accepts to carry, or even to become, something for which there is no theoretical remedy, something that cannot be digested, that resists being thought about, free associated to, or even dreamed about.

Presencing, withnessing and at-one-ment

As the reader will already have surmised, I think that the implications of this extraordinary moment, which Eshel captures so well, are obscured by uncritical acceptance of the now canonical language of O. This language helps us to evade the practical truth, which is that we do not have a technique and that our mentalistic model of the psyche is inadequate. As Eshel shows, what we like to call O involves something more heterogeneous, fluid, and dynamic than Bion's terms suggest; it is a chaotic process rather than a steady state of the analytic mind; it is more like a moment of incoherence, when the analytic "system" teeters on the brink of collapse into chaos.

This insight is clearly reflected in the final section of her first chapter (this volume), where Eshel emphasizes the element, in her own experience, of anomie, dissociation, blankness and paralysis. She hypothesizes from various perspectives that she had in effect allowed herself to become colonized by the whole of Clari's ongoing psychic calamity. I think this is exactly right. But at the same time, Ofra says that she did this "without dread." She experiences a kind of "vicarious dissociation" in which she is able psychically to embody for Clari, with Clari, a different way of experiencing the terrifyingly lonely "darkness":

> the experience of being inside a massive dissociative, blank process was occurring in *me—a vicarious self-state dissociation,* thus detaching and distancing it from her while she observed from without. But when I let it affect me, allowing it to be and become me, without understanding it but also without dread, carrying in me the knowledge from experience of having been repeatedly dissociated and absent—yet staying there, in the treatment, surviving, trying to hold and think the experience—it gradually became a therapeutic experience. The dissociation very slowly became a new kind of dissociation—*an attenuated, deferred dissociation,* because the dissociation in me—or, more precisely, in the interconnected entity of her-and-me—was no longer the extremely lonely, unmediated, life-defending dissociative self-experience of her,

> but a dissociative experience that was held differently within me, and within a human process—a massive yet sustained and tolerable one.[11]

As we can see from her manner of expression, Eshel's ideas about connecting with her patient are very different from the privileged metaphysical perspective of Bion's *Attention and Interpretation*. She uses an unassuming phrase: "the interconnected entity of her-and-me." This "her-and-me," joined with hyphens, strikes me as an apt way of putting what her concept of presencing actually involves: it creates or taps into a heterogeneous 'entity,' a sometimes almost teratoma-like thing, which includes the presence of the non-human, and even the inhuman—or the 'uncanny' as Freud liked to put it. In relation to another patient, a sex offender, Eshel refers to this aspect as 'chimeric,' or in other words, hybrid and monstrous (2019, pp. 92ff). The analytic relationship at this "deep level of interconnectedness" is not merely a dyad that can somehow be melded or distilled into an oceanic homogeneity. Presencing and withnessing in the meaningful practical sense are not like states of fusion in which, by definition, there can be no differentiation.

Without going into the semantic ingenuity of these terms, it is evident that presencing and withnessing bring out a latent aspect of the analyst's function, which is to place oneself in a position to be able to testify to the existence, the occurrence, the *event* of another's life and being. If pursued intrepidly, the combination of presencing and withnessing may deepen into 'at-onement' with the patient's innermost reality. In that sense, the interpsychic connection of presencing, withnessing, and at-one-ment that develops may be *as close as we can come to experiencing an other's "natality"* in Hannah Arendt's existential sense of that term. This would not be a psychoanalytically privileged state of mind that we can claim to professionally possess. Nor is it a primordial ethical demand in the Levinasian sense, something that we can deduce on philosophical first principles as a universal truth and then claim as the essence of psychoanalysis (cf. Chetrit-Vatine, 2018).

To be sure, when Eshel tries to convey how she connects with psychically very remote patients, she touches on an element that is implicit in the therapeutic aim of psychoanalysis—but this is not something we can claim hubristically as our foundation, as if it were built in to the way we work. Rather, it is a potential that we might discover in the process of doing psychoanalysis as we have otherwise come to understand it. In this perspective, presencing, withnessing, and at-one-ment are not automatically "interpellated" by the patient's suffering (or by O); they can only be achieved by means of a personal surrender that Eshel describes and redescribes from many different angles. In the kinds of clinical situation she brings to life for us in her writing, she captures a vital quality of sheer determination to somehow stay in the orbit of the patient, even as all the prescribed, often highly idealized, smoothly functioning analytic states of mind fail.

It is significant that Eshel frames her concepts of presencing, withnessing, and at-one-ment by distinguishing them from the concept of intersubjectivity as we understand it today in psychoanalysis. I think this goes hand in hand with my earlier suggestion that reverie and containment, which are linked to some of the higher forms of psychoanalytic intersubjectivity, are clinically restricted in the scope of inter-connection they actually permit. Eshel is pointing us to the limits of the analytic dyad, our convenient theoretical illusion of two subjects in an exclusive relationship that is believed to be therapeutically adequate (for a related perspective, see Tennes, 2007). In such an imaginary relationship, we would never need to leave the comfortable realm of conventional humanity to enter the wilderness of the non-human and the unknown; we would never need to acknowledge the weirdness of a world where disavowal and denial seem indispensable to a comfortable sense of self. In this sense, Martin Buber's "I-Thou" relationship is a deceptive idealization. If we accept the reality of unconscious forces in our lives, we cannot logically conceptualize the psychoanalytic relationship as merely a "two-person psychology." How can we truly stay in the presence of a patient like Clari, who is alone in the dark and wandering sightlessly in the desert, if we are not willing to be "eyeless in the Gaza Strip," to paraphrase Milton, and sit among the desolate ruins? What else but the inhuman would be so resistant to the efforts of our well-meaning, intersubjective techniques?

On subjectivity and the problem of the third

From this vantage, it is also noteworthy that Ofra rarely, if ever, uses the language of thirdness. The "third" in our current discourse has two dominant meanings. It began as a Kleinian euphemism for the limiting authority of the Oedipal father (the frame), as in the analyst's reliance on theory and training as a counterweight to the patient's transference demands (resistance). Analysts who adopt this perspective speak lovingly of being held and contained by psychoanalytic theory. The now more popular usage of triangularity is exemplified in field theory, or in Ogden's (1994) useful idea of the "intersubjective third" as a kind of interpsychic co-creation. For Eshel, this conceptualization of an enveloping thirdness depends, perhaps too heavily, on the input of the analyst's personal autobiographical subjectivity. In this respect, it is related to but somewhat different from the concept of 'chimera' in French psychoanalysis (M'Uzan, 1978, 1976). Eshel uses the same term in a more impersonal sense that is telling: she draws on the biomedical analogy of "chimeric antibodies that bind to the antigen to fight the pathogen, but without triggering the immune reaction in the body" (2019, p. 92). What she is saying, I think, is that in becoming the other of the patient, Eshel does not draw deliberately on associations and analogies to her own personal experience. Her manner of reaching the patient is not 'empathic' in the traditional sense of projecting the self into the other. It is more like what Deleuze and Guattari (1987) describe as "becoming animal."[12]

As Eshel points out, in our various theories of "enactment,"[13] we remain too dependent on the function of the analyst's personal subjectivity. We tend to conceptualize intersubjectivity as a relation of subject to subject, involving a method in which the analyst more or less self-consciously uses their own autobiographical memory as a channel into the patient's realm of experience (Jacobs, 1993; Ogden, 1994). Eshel provides us with a much more radical challenge: "I differ from Ogden," she says,

> in the emphasis he places on the analyst's own subjective past experiences and memories, which are evoked in the analyst's mind in the session. I reach out toward the analyst's embeddedness in the patient's subjective reality, especially as a necessary functioning presence, by … letting the patient's subjective reality impose itself … The analyst thus becomes part of the patient's state of being and experiencing, to the extent of becoming psychically akin to a transplant or to chimeric antibodies.
>
> (2019, p. 38)

Ofra's work implies for me that the whole lexicon of the countertransference revolution in psychoanalytic theory too easily turns into a reassuring strategy for keeping our clinical experience within the language of social propriety. Ofra points us to the area beyond the human subject and even beyond the self; she pulls us toward the furthest outreaches of sentience, even the inanimate, where intersubjectivity and reverie necessarily fail. It is worth noting that Bion in fact did describe O as a "non-human system" (Bion, 1970, p. 103; CW 6, p. 308). I would suggest that the possibility of the inhuman within us (not the same as 'barbarity,' which is eminently human) is one of the things that Freud intuited about the unconscious; it may have been what he was clumsily groping toward in his theory of the biological 'death instinct' (Freud, 1920). Unfortunately, clinical psychoanalysis has missed this insight, partly because Freud failed to theorize the transversal qualities of unconscious mental life. He opted instead to populate the unconscious with familiar family-like figures, through a kind of humanistic Lamarckianism, as in his reassuring theory of a nuclear Oedipus complex.

The contrast of this traditional view of the unconscious with Eshel's clinical work at the level of passionate inter-embodied experience is striking. It suggests to me that the classical Freudian unconscious (timelessness, exemption from the 'logic' of embodied experience, and thus, implicitly, *transcendence*) has unfortunately become a way of repackaging the unconscious to make it more palatable to the public, the insurance companies, and of course, ourselves. This 'transcendental' unconscious is now the source of a most admirable "truth drive" (Grotstein, 2007, p. 52)—how could anyone object to that? It seems that something like this kind of idealization of the psyche has been going on in the creative use we have been making of Bion's idiosyncratic vocabulary. In this perspective, the high-sounding language of O, negative capability, and so on, as designating a realm of truth-in-being unsullied by the body ("with no sensuous background") lends itself to be used as a euphemistic public relations language; it provides a verbal cover for experimenting with "intersubjectivity" and other forms of relationality that would not otherwise have been sanctionable by the central psychoanalytic authorities (and were not within Bion's original purview). It can also be used to distract attention from the otherwise unfathomable contingencies of working beyond the reach of any discernible method. Phrases like 'to be at one' with the patient and "to become 'O'" provide deceptively reassuring ways of verbally finessing the fact that in moments of criticality in the psychoanalytic process, when everything is tipping toward potential chaos (Bion's catastrophic change [CW 5, pp. 132–134]), we actually have no idea what we are doing, and there is no way to understand what is happening (even in retrospect, assuming it turns out well) in terms of our existing developmental and psychodynamic theories.

That psychoanalysis can be dangerous and perhaps even 'perverse' in this way—that in the pursuit of its aims it may require something like what Saketopoulou (2023) has described as the "traumato*philic*" risk-taking of "limit consent"—is not something that our profession is happy to make explicit in public discourse.[14] Till now, psychoanalytic transcendentalism, especially of the Bionian sort (an appealing variant of essentialism), has provided many of us with a convenient alibi for covert explorations of these issues. From the perspective of clinical innovation under the aegis of the psychoanalytic Establishment (Bion, 1970, pp. 62–124; CW 6, pp. 273–326), this has been a good thing so far as it goes. One can sometimes stay under the radar by invoking the Messiah in whose name the Establishment functions. But it seems to me that the cumulative effects of Eshel's brilliant case discussions have been to blow our professional cover.

Another way to understand this point would be in terms of Greenberg's (2015) proposition about our different theories of therapeutic action. If he is right that the latter are essentially "controlling fictions" (pp. 17ff) that govern our sense of what to do in the analytic process, then we might speculate that what Dr. Eshel does, in the moments of criticality we are considering, is simply to let what happens tell the story, if that is possible.[15] In any case, I think she really does take us into the wilderness—the formidable "venture zone." Where within the psychoanalytic canon of technique can we find a match for her willingness to be slipped into a state of practical oblivion? In Bion's attempts to "dream" the session, he often worried about falling asleep (CW 11, p. 83; Bion, 1970, p. 47 [CW 6, p. 260]); and even Winnicott (1962, p. 166) assumed as a rule the imperative to stay awake during the session

Part 3. The problem of unconscious communication

If what happened with Clari in some ways challenges the axiom that the analyst must be conscious while working, we find ourselves face to face with the vexing question of unconscious communication, the rather vague term we use for an undoubted fact of material life in psychoanalysis. Dr. Eshel's work can be read as a practical guide to the problem of unconscious communication, and I believe we can best understand her approach in the framework of what I earlier called the theory of the embodied mind. This approach has three important aspects consistent with Eshel's work.

The first is the need for psychoanalysis to wean itself off the concept of "representation," especially when we are speaking of symbolization. In actuality we are bathing in unconscious symbolic processes all the time—through these unconscious processes, we live, breathe, create, and destroy. The psyche is not a "representational world" separate from our physical being. What we call the unconscious is precisely our embodied environment, swirling around us like an elemental medium upon which our existence materially depends. The unconscious in this sense refuses the binary logic of container and contained. The psyche is embodied, embedded in contingency, and extended beyond the conventional boundaries of the organism; and perhaps most importantly, it is enacted from the bottom up, barely depending upon our conscious awareness. The symbolic process needs to be approached, therefore, as an idiomatic singularity that cannot be captured in the theoretical language of representation, or for that matter, the "unrepresented." Winnicott often spoke of the infant's "imaginative elaboration of bodily experience." This phrase captures my understanding of what we mean by the term psychic life: it does not necessarily need to be "represented," or "mentalized;" and it is certainly not "represented" by symbols: it *is* the symbolic process itself, and it necessarily circulates via the media of otherness (Levin, 1989, 2003).

The idea that symbolization is the substance of the psyche, not its mere representation, has enormous implications for our conception of the psychoanalytic relationship. For example, it obviates the classical theory of resistance. Dr Eshel's clinical work illustrates this beautifully. For her, I believe, it is the analyst's resistance that needs to be overcome, not the patient's. Her falling asleep in Clari's presence is a good example; she had to overcome her own resistance—to cross her internal Rubicon—in order to connect. In that sense, Eshel's sleeping in the session can be understood, paradoxically, as her psychic surrender to Clari. Of course, Clari may not have understood this, and it is interesting to speculate why she tolerated Eshel's unusual clinical gesture. I suspect that it may have had something to do with what Eshel elsewhere describes (2019, pp. 112–113; 189), citing Ettinger, as "fascinance" in the primordial matrixial space, a kind of infant wonderment at the existential beauty of the mother, which Meltzer (Meltzer and Harris, 1988) has also explored in terms of the infant's original 'aesthetic conflict.' What Eshel's sleep may have symbolized for Clari, in the embodied sense of that term, was profound maternal peace. In any case, Clari did not ultimately construe Eshel's sleeping as a personal rejection, in spite of Eshel's seeming reluctance to work with her. At a level that counted, Clari must have understood the underlying logic of radical surrender, and was thus enabled, gradually, to surrender herself. A reciprocal inter-embodied process may have been at work, and I would love to know more of Eshel's thoughts on this possibility.

The need to relate to the patient's psychic life as an embodied experience—as a whole "pattern of being" (Gallagher, 2024)—leads us to the second aspect of unconscious communication, namely, the paradox that we can only be in unconscious contact so long as we are able to suspend the question whether we are dealing with our own unconscious or the unconscious of the other. For all we know, we may be dealing with a social unconscious that inhabits us, as in the paradigmatic example of the holocaust and its endless repetition in ordinary social and political life, even in our supposedly safe democracies today. In that sense, an unconscious connection is rather like Winnicott's transitional object—it is only "real" if it is left undecidable (Winnicott, 1971). What Eshel shows us is that the analyst's acceptance of this indeterminacy is fundamental to working at the level of the embodied mind. Nevertheless, this can be threatening to our professional identity; it may pull us in many directions that we are afraid to go.

The problem of undecidability takes us to a third paradox of unconscious communication, namely, that we only become aware of our unconscious connection with the patient when the connection falters or breaks down. We might analogize this to a crisis in the status of transitional object experience: is it me or not me—must I decide? Sometimes the analyst may suddenly realize that they were not as connected to the patient as they had assumed. At other times, they discover that they have been more connected than they had dared to hope.

One of the interesting aspects of Eshel's work with Clari is that their lack of connection was in many ways the central feature of their relationship, starting with the fact that Eshel was initially reluctant to take Clari on as a patient, and vice versa. The therapeutic relationship began with an ongoing relational impasse at the practical level, involving many delays; these delays continued into the later period of transition to more frequent sessions, the quantitative transition from psychotherapy to psychoanalysis. In her account of the analysis, Eshel is matter of fact about these significant disjunctions, even at the personal level, between herself and Clari.

That Eshel highlights the discontinuities in the relationship is salient. To me it suggests that she is pointing us to practical realities of presencing and withnessing that are not accounted for in conventional theories of attunement. My understanding is that she has her own intuitive way, which cannot be mummified into a technical precept, of connecting with her patients even at the point of maximum disconnection. In this way, at the level of inter-embodied presence, she can remain unconsciously in touch with a mind whose orientation is radically dissociative.

In the paper "Violent Innocence," Christopher Bollas brilliantly captured this paradox. He wrote, "It is likely that we are compelled to know more about the other when the illusion of understanding breaks down" (1992, p. 187). In saying this, Bollas was not trying to make a virtue out of not understanding; he was highlighting the importance of our capacity to recognize and accept when the *illusion* of unconscious interconnectedness, necessary for social communication, fails. On this view, psychoanalysis is not best described in terms of 'identification' or attunement; it is about finding ways to connect when the more or less normal feeling of like-mindedness has become practically unattainable. It is precisely this that is pathognomonic, making withnessing and presencing so necessary. Such may be the essence of psychoanalytic action: how one handles the impossibility of communication with any particular patient.

Inspired by Eshel's clinical studies, I have been describing the spirit of psychoanalytic practice as a form of inter-embodied psychic action. What do I mean by this phrase? Winnicott's (1971) answer was 'play,' but this is not so easy as it sounds. Bollas captured some of the implications in the following observation:

> Because we do not comprehend one another we are free to misperceive—in an act of creativity—and so, out of the gap emerges unconscious mental life, or intersubjective play, which brings us closer together. We do not thoughtfully understand one another any better … but as we play we come closer to one another
>
> (1992, pp. 186–187)

I like Bollas' formulation, but Eshel takes us further. She shows us that play in psychoanalysis is not only an expression of psychic freedom, but can also be an existentially bewildering necessity. If inter-embodied psychic action is play, in psychoanalysis it may have to be more than personal spontaneity; it may also involve a possible submission to the invasive logic of the other; a willingness to enter into a terrible game in which the rules are set by the patient's narcissistic demands, and may suddenly be changed without notice.[16]

Bollas links the possibility of unconscious communication to the psychic freedom to misperceive the other. All of Eshel's case discussions illustrate this existential paradox in working with what we call the unconscious—or in promoting its possible coming into being. She captures the essence of Winnicott's implicit message that when it actually counts, we have no recourse to a particular method. But then she takes us a step beyond, even further into the wilderness: she demonstrates that we have no recourse to a privileged psychoanalytic state of mind either, what many of us still feel Bion promised. We are always dealing with the practical undecidability of the unconscious we are trying to connect with. All we have to work with is pragmatic acceptance of the patient as other, as perhaps ontologically different, as fundamentally uninterpretable. We try to cope with how this otherness may move us in directions that we cannot anticipate. In this way, we hope to imagine, and thus personally embody, as it were in holographic fashion (Grotstein, 1979, p. 145), the other's mind.

Eshel's going to sleep illustrates the complexity of embodied relatedness. The quality of her sleep was featureless and dreamless—but it was still symbolic, at the most elemental level, beyond the scope of alpha function or beta elements. If we think of it in developmental time, her sleep suggests an imaginary moment in bodily existence, a sort of elemental proprioception, prior to sensing one's own physical being, as symbolized in Clari's persistent imagery of total darkness. Clari was eventually able to provide some relevant etiological history for this, but we are not in a position to understand precisely how Clari's way of being came about. In Eshel's descent into the paradoxical states that her surrender to Clari induced, she was not playing with Clari as one subject in spontaneous exchange with another subject, nor was she in a state of "evenly suspended attention"; nor was she indulging herself in an exotic form of social exchange. Her capacity for inter-embodied psychic action is frankly mysterious and, in my opinion, it should remain so. We should not be too self-conscious in the attempt to imitate her, because her way of connecting to her patients is so dependent on contingency, and so open to singularities—phenomena that are unpredictable and unrepeatable. Nevertheless, the examples she offers provide us with a unique psychoanalytic affordance. Hopefully, we can internalize them, without having to objectify her deep clinical wisdom into another professional dogma.

Notes

1 Versions of this paper were presented in Montreal, May, 2023, at the Quebec English Branch of the Canadian Psychoanalytic Society, and in Los Angeles, March 29, 2025, at the New Center for Psychoanalysis.

2 The terms "critical and pastoral knowledge interests (or aims) of psychoanalysis" refer to a fundamental tension within Freud's psychoanalytic project. 'Critical' refers broadly to Freud's scientific-epistemological aspirations for psychoanalysis. 'Pastoral' refers to Freud's interest in healing, his various therapeutic ideas and strategies. Contrary to Freud's original hopes, the critical and pastoral aims of psychoanalysis frequently conflict.

3 Freud (1933, p. 80) used the image of reclaiming dry land from the "oceanic" realm, as in the draining of the Zuider Zee: "where id was, there ego shall be."

4 There is a sense in which Freud positioned the practice of psychoanalysis somewhere between the interests and perspectives of the infantile body and those of civilization. As I have argued (Levin, 2000), psychoanalysis implies a kind of liminal sub-culture—a culture of 'acivilization.'

5 For further discussion of this complex question, see my forthcoming book, A Critical Companion to Bion: Functions of a Psychoanalytic Personality. New York: Routledge, 2026. See also Eshel (2022).

6 The earlier published Brazilian lectures and consultations can be found in volumes 7 and 8 of Bion's Collected Works (Bion, 2014), henceforth referred to in the text as CW followed by the volume number.

7 In an illuminating discussion of Bion's evolution as an analyst, Eshel (2022) has tried to situate these features of Bion's clinical work in the broader context of his innovative contribution.

8 Ecological is relating to or concerned with the relation of living organisms to one another and to their physical environment.

9 The philosopher Thomas Nagel (2024) has pointed out that, for good reasons, "the conceptual scheme of our natural language is dualistic" (p. 31). However, he also argues in favour of the idea that

> in spite of what our natural language concepts seem to imply, the truth lies in some form of monism … that conscious mental properties and their neurophysiological conditions are not distinct but are inseparable aspects of some one thing, for which we do not at present have a concept.
>
> (pp. 34–35)

No doubt Bion's all-embracing vision of ultimate reality as O sprang from a similar intuition.

10 "With each birth something uniquely new comes into the world" (Arendt, 1958, p. 178). Arendt anchored the elements of the human condition, including plurality and sociability, in natality, that is, in recognition of the essential freedom, creativity and innovation implied in every new beginning of a distinct human life.
11 There is a striking passage in Bion's description of the effects of cultivating the suppression of memory and desire where one might find a link to Eshel's falling asleep, though it differs in key respects from her description of that process. Bion wrote: "The nearer the analyst comes to achieving suppression of desire, memory, and understanding, *the more likely he is to slip into a sleep akin to stupor*. Though different, the difference is hard to define. The sharpening of contact with O cannot be separated from an increase of perception, in particular of elements of K; this sensuous sharpening is painful although partial and mitigated by the general obliteration of sensory perception. The residual sensory perception, often auditory and restricted to particular kinds of sound, is responsible for inducing a sharp and painful reaction (similar to the startle reaction seen in babies)" (1970, p. 47; 2014, CW 6, p. 260, emphasis added).
12 In the phrase 'becoming animal,' Deleuze and Guattari offered an Ovidian evocation of unconscious psychic life as a form of otherness that participates, impersonally and non-hierarchically, in unpredictable affiliations with the multiplicity of all beings, living or otherwise. Their provocative way of reframing the unconscious in a less recognizably human guise than Freud proposed may resonate with readers who appreciate Bion's later work.
13 For an illuminating study of this concept, see Katz (2014).
14 Saketopoulou states: "In contrast to affirmative consent, limit consent hinges not on respecting limits but on their ethical transgression. Limit consent runs on nonlinear time, blurs the divide between active and passive, and comes dangerously close to the line of something going wrong" (Saketopoulou, 2023, p. 58; see also, "Consent in the Psychoanalytic Situation," pp. 65–68 in the same work).
15 Greenberg states that "certainly there is no way to step outside our narrative structure to conceptualize a sequence of events that has led to benign change" (p. 22).
16 I appreciate Ghent's (1990) distinction between submission and surrender, but prefer to keep the word submission here, despite its connotations of masochistic perversity.

References

Aguayo, J. & Malin, B. (2013). *Wilfrid Bion: Los Angeles Seminars and Supervision*. New York and London: Routledge.

Aguayo, J., Pistiner de Cortinas, L. & Regeczkey (eds.) (2018). *Bion in Buenos Aires: Seminars, Case Presentation, and Supervision*. London and New York: Routledge.

Arendt, H. (1958). *The Human Condition.* Chicago: University of Chicago Press.

Beckett, S. (1965). *Three Novels by Samuel Becket: Molloy, Malone Dies, The Unnamable.* New York: Grove Press.

Benjamin, W. (1969). Theses on the philosophy of history. In H. Zohn (trans.), *Illuminations* (p. 249). New York: Schocken Books.

Bion, W. R. (1970). *Attention and Interpretation.* London: Tavistock.

Bion, W. R. (1980). *Bion in New York and Sao Paulo.* Ed. F. Bion. Pertshire: Clunie Press.

Bion, W. R. (1991). *A Memoir of the Future.* London: Karnac.

Bion, W. R. (2014). *The Complete Works of W.R. Bion.* C.Mawson (Ed). London and New York: Routledge.

Bollas, C. (1992). Violent innocence. In *Being a Character: Psychoanalysis and Self-Experience* (pp. 165–192). NewYork: Hill and Wang.

Carhart-Harris, R. & Friston, K. (2010). The default-mode, ego functions and free-energy: A neurological account of Freudian ideas. *Brain,* 133: 1265–1283.

Chetrit-Vatine, V. (2018). *The Ethical Seduction of the Analytic Situation: The Feminine-Maternal Origins of Responsibility for the Other.* Trans. A. Weller. New York and London: Routledge.

Civitarese, G. (2025). We-community, *Ineinandersein* and intersubjectivity in psychoanalysis: Notes in the margin of *Husserl's Legacy*, by Dan Zahavi. *Psychoanalytic Inquiry*, 45(3): 281294. (Published online, April 2025). https://doi.org/10.1080/07351690.2025.2476899.

Clark, A. (2023). *The Experience Machine. How our minds predict and shape reality.* New York: Random.

Deleuze, G. & Guattari, F. (1987). *A Thousand Plateaus: Capitalism and Schizophrenia.* Trans. B. Massumi. Minneapolis: University of Minnesota Press.

Eshel, O. (2004). "Green woman" to "scheherazade": The becoming of a fundamentally new experience in psychoanalytic treatment. *Contemporary Psychoanalysis*, 40(4): 527–556.

Eshel, O. (2019). *The Emergence of Analytic Oneness: Into the Heart of Psychoanalysis.* New York: Routledge.

Eshel, O. (2022). Bion's long road toward intuiting the patient's suffering: 'Theoretical' vs. 'clinical' Bion. *Contemporary Psychoanalysis*, 58: 46–76.

Freud, S. (1920). Beyond the pleasure principle. *The Complete Psychological Works of Sigmund Freud*, 18: 7–66.

Freud, S. (1933). The new introductory lectures. *The Complete Psychological Works of Sigmund Freud*, 22: 5–182.

Gallagher, S. (2005). *How the Body Shapes the Mind.* Oxford: Clarendon Press.

Gallagher, S. (2024). *The Self and its Disorders.* Oxford: Oxford University Press.

Ghent, E. (1990). Masochism, submission, surrender—Masochism as a perversion of surrender. *Contemporary Psychoanalysis* 26: 108–136.

Greenberg, J. (2015). Therapeutic action and the analyst's responsibility. *Journal of the American Psychoanalytic Association,* 63(1): 15–32.

Grotstein, J. (2007). *A Beam of Intense Darkness: Wilfred Bion's Legacy to Psychoanalysis.* London: Karnac.

Grotstein, J. S. (1979). Who is the dreamer who dreams the dream and who is the dreamer who understands it—A psychoanalytic inquiry into the ultimate nature of being. *Contemporary Psychoanalysis*, 15: 110–169.

Habermas, J. (1972). *Knowledge and Human Interests*. Trans. J. Shapiro. Boston, MA: Beacon Press.

Jacobs, T. J. (1993). The inner experiences of the analyst: Their contribution to the analytic process. *International Journal of Psychoanalysis*, 74: 7–14.

Katz, G. (2014). *The Play Within the Play: The Enacted Dimension of Psychoanalytic Process*. New York: Routledge.

Kirschner, L. (ed) (2011). *Between Winnicott and Lacan: A Clinical Engagement*. New York: Routledge.

Levin, C. (1989). *An Essay on the Symbolic Process*. Ph.D. thesis. Department of Humanities, Concordia University, Montreal.

Levin, C. (2000). Le devenir d'une acivilization. In D. Scarfone (ed.), *L'Avenir d'une désillusion* (pp. 99–117). Paris: P.U.F.

Levin, C. (2003). Containing the container: Some experiential aspects of narcissism and the problem of "primary undifferentiation." *Israel Psychoanalytic Journal*, 1(2): 167–202.

Meltzer, D. (1981). The Kleinian expansion of Freud's metapsychology. *International Journal of Psychoanalysis*, 62: 177–185.

Meltzer, D. & Harris, M. (1988). *The Apprehension of Beauty*. Pertshire: Clunie Press.

M'Uzan, M. d. (1976). Countertransference and the paradoxical system. In A. Weller (trans.), *Death and Identity: Being and the psycho-sexual drama* (pp. 16–32). London/New York: Routledge, 2018.

M'Uzan, M. d. (1978). La bouche de l'inconscient. *Nouvelle Revue de Psychanalyse*, 17: 89–98.

Nagel, T. (2024). Further thoughts: The psychophysical nexus. In *What Is It Like to Be a Bat?* (pp. 31–53). Oxford: Oxford University Press.

Ogden, T. H. (1994). The analytic third: Working with intersubjective clinical facts. *International Journal of Psychoanalysis*, 75(1): 3–19.

Ogden, T. H. (2019). Ontological psychoanalysis or "what do you want to be when you grow up?" *Psychoanalytic Quarterly*, 88: 661–684.

Saketopoulou, A. (2023). *Sexuality Beyond Consent: Risk, Race, Traumatophilia*. New York: New York University Press.

Solms, M. (2023). *The Hidden Spring: A Journey to the Source of Consciousness*. New York: Norton.

Tennes, M. (2007). Beyond intersubjectivity: The transpersonal dimension of the psychoanalytic encounter. *Contemporary Psychoanalysis*, 43(4): 505–525.

Varela, F., Thompson, E. & Rosch, E. (2016). *The Embodied Mind: Cognitive Science and Human Experience*. Revised Edition. Cambridge, MA: MIT Press. (Originally published 1991).

Winnicott, D. W. (1949). Mind and its relation to the psyche-soma. In *Through Pediatrics to Psychoanalysis* (pp. 243–254). New York: Basic Books, 1975.
Winnicott, D. W. (1962). The aims of the psycho-analytical treatment. In *The Maturational Processes and the Facilitating Environment: Studies in the Theory of Emotional Development* (pp. 166–170). New York: International Universities Press, 1965.
Winnicott, D. W. (1971). *Playing and Reality*. Harmondworth: Penguin.

Chapter 3

Fascinated and troubled in contemporary psychoanalysis

Ofra Eshel's extension of the Bion-Winnicott framework for working with severe traumatic states

Aner Govrin

Characteristics of fascinated and troubled communities

This chapter is divided into two parts. In the first part, I present the theory I developed in my book *Conservative and Radical Perspectives on Psychoanalytic Knowledge: The Fascinated and the Disenchanted* (2015), which outlines two types of psychoanalytic communities: **fascinated communities** and **troubled communities.**

In the second part, I put forward my main thesis: I aim to situate Ofra Eshel's role within this framework. I describe her as a *fascinated–troubled* analyst—an analyst with a clear identity who aligns with the fascinated community of Bion and Winnicott, while at the same time contributing significant innovations from within this community, beyond Bion and Winnicott.

Psychoanalysis, it might be said, was not supposed to exist today. Until recently, many indicators suggested it was on the verge of extinction. After all, it has endured numerous setbacks: it has long been met with contempt and hostility from academic psychology, since few of its concepts have strong empirical support. Psychoanalysis has been repeatedly eulogized by critics and even by some of its supporters, who predicted its inevitable demise.

Yet these predictions have proven dramatically wrong. Just a few decades after fears of its extinction, psychoanalytic theory is experiencing a remarkable resurgence. In recent years, it has become richer and more diverse, enjoying an exciting period of intellectual and clinical renewal as it continues to generate new theories about the human mind. Around the world, vibrant psychoanalytic communities persist—believing in it,

DOI: 10.4324/9781003674078-5

developing it, and practicing it as a treatment method. In fact, psychoanalysis has become one of the most enduring intellectual enterprises in Western thought, remarkable both for its ability to build a body of knowledge and for its longevity. It continues to thrive, showing no signs of decline. This raises a crucial question: What enables the psychoanalytic community to withstand such persistent criticism and hostility? Is its success merely the result of loyal followers who isolate themselves within theoretical schools? Or does psychoanalysis possess healthy mechanisms that promote growth and self-renewal? Has it adapted to our changing world and responded effectively to modern challenges over the years?

In my 2015 book (Govrin, 2015), I argue that the dynamic interplay between loyalty and criticism has kept psychoanalysis alive. Mechanisms of deep commitment on the one hand and of doubt, questioning, and skepticism on the other, as well as the *tensions* between them, have preserved its vitality. Throughout its history, psychoanalysis has managed to combine what I call *fascinated communities* and *troubled communities*. This blend accounts for its longevity, its rich diversity, and its ability to continue attracting new generations of therapists. Similar processes can be observed in other scientific traditions. For a theory to survive, it requires a loyal following that believes in it, experiences it as true, and develops it with passion. Inevitably, the theory encounters critique—its weaknesses, paradoxes, and failures are exposed. Sometimes, it collapses and is replaced. At other times, it adapts and expands in multiple directions, becoming richer and more nuanced.

It is this tension between the theory and its criticism, between the loyalists and the skeptics, that fuels change, development, and deepening. The friction is a source of vitality and resilience. Thanks to it, psychoanalysis is not abandoned, nor do its adherents sink into complacency. Instead, they innovate and keep it relevant. The dialectic between fascination and trouble allows renewal to emerge even amid criticism, hostility, and contempt.

Let us now turn to the two types of communities more closely. A **fascinated community** is a group for whom one psychoanalytic theory (for example, those of Klein, Bion, Kohut, or Winnicott) becomes an all-encompassing worldview. Paraphrasing Pepper (1942) and Freud (1933), one could say that fascinated communities treat a given theory as a worldview that explains all forms of human distress as part of a unified system. Within such a framework, every significant aspect of human behavior finds its place, and every clinical problem appears explicable within a single coherent set of principles. The theory promises unlimited applicability—an alluring completeness that makes it feel as though it can explain everything. In practice, no psychoanalytic school—or scientific theory—ever fulfills such an ideal. Yet this promise of wholeness is part of what gives fascinated communities their magnetic power.

An instructive historical example can be found in the history of the Los Angeles Psychoanalytic Society and Institute (LAPSI), as described by the Australian scholar Douglas Kirsner in his book *Unfree Associations*. The visits of leading Kleinians to Los Angeles in the 1970s—Herbert Rosenfeld, Wilfred Bion, Albert Mason, Hanna Segal, Betty Joseph, and Donald Meltzer—sparked tremendous excitement and a sense of revelation. The Kleinians were perceived as bearers of the truth, with Rosenfeld, for instance, being compared to Moses descending from Mount Sinai with the tablets of the covenant. At the same time, however, the Kleinian approach met fierce resistance from within the institute. In fact, LAPSI housed two types of fascinated communities, each hostile to the other: those loyal to Klein and those loyal to Freud. The tension between these factions reached a climax when the national organization intervened and demanded the expulsion of all Kleinians from the institute.

This episode shows how dangerous fascinated communities can become. Yet my book is, to a large extent, a defense of fascinated communities that work passionately to develop and deepen their theories from within. Thanks to them, psychoanalysis continues to exist. Without fascinated communities, we would not still be studying, teaching, and rereading Freud, Klein, Winnicott, Bion, or Lacan; nor would we be organizing conferences, journals, workshops, and training institutes dedicated to their thought.

Indeed, can any meaningful human project—from raising children through creating art to cultivating a garden—be sustained without fascination? The same holds true for scientific and psychoanalytic endeavors. However, fascination alone can easily slide into dogma. It can continue to inspire creativity only when troubled communities exist and remain active alongside it.

Thus, fascinated communities have several defining characteristics. They diligently preserve their original ideas, and changes within them occur only gradually over many years. Most of the concepts developed by Klein, Bion, Lacan, Winnicott, and Kohut—such as *projective identification*, *reverie*, *transitional object*, *mirror stage*, and *transmuting internalization*—remain central to community members today. These communities are devoted to rereading and reinterpreting the same foundational texts—by Freud, Jung, Lacan, Bion, Klein, Kohut, and others—that define their school. While the texts themselves remain unchanged, their meanings evolve over time and acquire new significance. The key figures in fascinated communities are analysts who write about and interpret these canonical works, offering their colleagues innovative ways to apply existing theories—for example, Hanna Segal for Klein, Leon Gtinberg for Bion, Paul and Anna Ornstein or Arnold Goldberg for Kohut. Another trait of fascinated communities concerns their conception of truth. They tend to hold worldview perspectives akin to those of scientists, emphasizing realism and the correspondence theory of truth. Thus, the Kleinian community believes the infant is truly engaged in the fantasy of tearing the breast, the Kohutian community deeply believes in a *grandiose self*; and the Winnicottian community holds to the reality of an early stage in which the infant experiences itself as omnipotent.

Troubled communities, by contrast, challenge conventional thinking and create new research traditions. While fascinated communities continue to refine and deepen their existing frameworks, troubled communities embody the demand for change, critique, and the search for better alternatives to prevailing theories.

Despite their devotion, fascinated communities cannot sustain an entire discipline indefinitely. Their weakness lies in their being isolated—they tend to communicate only within their own circle, remain closed to external influences, and often fall out of touch with developments in science, philosophy, society, and culture. Over time, this isolation risks rendering them less relevant.

The major paradigmatic shifts in the history of psychoanalysis should therefore be attributed to troubled communities. The most familiar of these are those that founded new psychoanalytic schools. Their founders—Klein, Lacan, Bion, Winnicott, Kohut, and others—were analysts dissatisfied with existing theories of the human psyche. They developed new, comprehensive frameworks within the broader psychoanalytic community to address the limitations they perceived. For instance, Kohut observed that patients responded better to empathic understanding than to drive-based interpretation, and Klein sought to understand the destructive impulses of her young patients expressed in sadistic play.

Every fascinated community thus originates in a *troubled analyst*, joined by others who gather to reshape the body of knowledge. Over time, these analysts coalesce around shared problems, interventions, therapeutic goals, and conceptions of transference, forming a unified school. Eventually, such communities cease to be troubled; they become captivated by the comprehensive theories they themselves have created.

There are, however, other kinds of troubled communities besides those that establish new schools:

1. Scientific troubled communities—groups of researchers dedicated to studying psychodynamic therapeutic processes through empirical methods, such as Sidney Blatt, Jonathan Shedler, Mark Solms, and Beatrice Beebe.
2. Philosophically and culturally troubled communities—groups influenced by contemporary philosophical and cultural movements in the West, seeking to reconfigure psychoanalysis accordingly. The most prominent of these is the *relational approach*.

It is important to note that troubled analysts also exist within fascinated communities and play a vital role in their development. These analysts are stirred by a particular conceptual or technical problem within the existing framework and seek ways to resolve it. For example, Antonino Ferro's creative extensions of Bion's ideas demonstrate such internal innovation. The basic assumption, then, is that rather than dividing the psychoanalytic world into fascinated and troubled communities, we should understand it as a *dialectical movement* within the communities themselves—an ongoing oscillation between fascination and trouble. I would now like to connect all this to Ofra Eshel's ideas.

The transformative psychoanalytic vision of Ofra Eshel: beyond Bion and Winnicott

Ofra Eshel's therapeutic approach is remarkable for a key reason: her profound conviction that treatment can transform any patient, even those facing the most severe psychic challenges. This transformation becomes possible when analysts/therapists forge genuine, deep connections with their patients' emotional worlds. Eshel articulates this view across many of her papers and most comprehensively in her book *The Emergence of Analytic Oneness* (2019a).

What may sound simple in theory becomes far more complex in practice. Through Eshel's writings, it becomes evident that such transformation requires deliberate effort, profound experiential presence, attentive listening, and very deep attunement.

It also requires something even more radical from the analyst/therapist: a willingness to be vulnerable—to surrender to another's suffering and to experience its painful impacts within oneself. This connection manifests as direct experiential contact, emotional tangibility, and a wide-open heart, ready for feeling pain, sustaining it, and even transforming it into a "magical sensitivity" that can revive and meet the most primitive traumas and catastrophes within the therapeutic relatedness.

The origins of Eshel's theoretical innovation

Eshel's groundbreaking contributions to psychoanalytic theory and practice emerge from her deep engagement with the works of Donald Winnicott and Wilfred Bion (2015, 2017, 2019a, 2019b). Her innovations neither replicate nor merely synthesize their ideas but extend them in *radically new directions*.

Eshel's work addresses the central challenge of treating patients suffering from early breakdowns, mental catastrophic states, and unrepresented traumas—that seem beyond the reach of traditional analytic methods.

Winnicott, in his theory of regression, described the hope that treatment could offer a new opportunity for the frozen early states of maternal failure to thaw and be re-experienced within the analytic holding environment. But in his posthumously published work, he went even further, developing a radical understanding of early breakdown as the result of massive traumatic environmental failure. The agony of early breakdown, Winnicott suggested, is so unthinkable that it cannot be experienced, and a primitive defensive organization, manifesting as the patient's illness syndrome, shuts down the experience of intolerable agony. Thus, the buried, unexperienced trauma becomes a continuing catastrophic impact on one's being—that can only be transformed if it is *relived and experienced* within the analytic relationship.

In Bion's late writings, we find the radical idea that the analyst must be willing to abandon memory and desire to embody the patient's innermost psychic reality (O)—that cannot be known but only "become."

Eshel's work takes these profound ideas and develops them into a comprehensive clinical framework that tackles the most challenging aspects of working with severe traumatic and catastrophic psychic realities.

Eshel's core concepts

Hinachechut (presencing)

At the heart of Eshel's therapeutic approach lies the concept of *Hinachechut* (Eshel, 2019a)—derived in Hebrew from the combination of *nochechut* ("presence" or "deep availability") and *hinatnut* ("surrender" or "giving oneself over"). It designates the analyst's or therapist's willingness and ability to emotionally surrender to the grip of the analytic process, entering into direct contact with the patient's emotional reality and traumatic experience.

Hinachechut goes beyond empathy or attunement. It is an active state of being *within* the patient's experiential reality, allowing the analyst to experience and feel the patient's pain, suffering, shame, despair, and terror as they emerge—thus enabling analyst and patient to go through these experiences t(w)ogether in a profound psyche-to-psyche connection.

Interconnectedness and withness

Eshel introduces the ideas of "interconnectedness" and "withness" (a term that is **essentially** different from *witness*) to highlight the analyst's deep, living connection with the patient. The analyst does not simply observe or testify to the patient's experience but **joins and shares** it. This is not merely an intersubjective relationship between two subjects; it transcends usual boundaries to form what Eshel (2019a) calls a "two-in-oneness," which may deepen into **at-one-ment** with the patient's innermost emotional reality. Thus, the analyst commits to becoming part of the patient's ongoing emotional reality and mental processes. Patient and analyst "**live** an experience together" (Winnicott, 1945), or, as Eshel (2019b) adds, "live the unthinkable, the unexperienced, and the unlived t(w)ogether" when working through extremely dark, unknown processes in challenging treatments.

Quantum interconnectedness

To illuminate the profound significance of this experience, Eshel borrows physicist David Bohm's notion of "the quantum interconnectedness of distant systems." This metaphor from quantum physics helps express how analyst and patient can become linked in ways that exceed traditional notions of separate subjectivities (Eshel, 2019a).

Just as in modern physics quantum mechanics introduced principles of uncertainty and the inseparability of observer and observed, in Eshel's view, analyst and patient can reach a state of non-separable wholeness that enables in-depth therapeutic transformation.

The spectrum of analytic oneness

Perhaps Eshel's most significant theoretical contribution is her concept of "the spectrum of analytic oneness." Although the term *oneness* has appeared in earlier psychoanalytic writings, Eshel's innovation lies in describing a **spectrum** of varying degrees of patient-analyst oneness that occur within different unconscious or unrepresented layers of experience that do not ordinarily communicate in analytic work.

This spectrum centers on the degree of **traumatization** and the **distortion or breakdown of basic processes of relatedness**, where representation is disrupted, regressively lost, or fails to develop altogether. At the same time, this conceptualization opens **new ontological and experiential (rather than epistemological)** possibilities for analytic work with the most difficult and fragmented psychic realities (Eshel, 2023).

The "hearing heart" and beyond representation

Eshel presents the powerful metaphor of the "hearing heart" ("Lev Shomea" in Hebrew), inspired by the biblical story of King Solomon asking God for a "hearing heart" to be able to judge his people. While standard translations of the Bible into English often call this "an understanding mind," Eshel emphasizes the deeper implication: the capacity to listen and understand with one's heart, not just the mind.

For Eshel, the heart is what hears the cry of trauma or the silenced, annihilated plea of breakdown. This is especially important when dealing with the "last scream" (Winnicott) or "unheard SOS" (Eigen) from the depths of catastrophic processes that began long ago and still go on. The analyst's heart can listen and "experience again and again the heartbreak that is at the center of human existence." This allows for a different way to reach and connect with the patient, experiencing the intensity and pain of heartbreak deep within the psyche.

The ability to have a "hearing heart" arises only when one is brave enough to open oneself vulnerably to another's experience. This is the core challenge for the analyst—often an extremely difficult one—to surrender completely, with "all one's heart, soul, might" (Eigen, 1981, based on Deuteronomy 6:5), inhabiting fully the patient's troubled emotional world. It requires maintaining an open, receptive stance while sensing, hearing, and feeling the patient's trauma or breakdown as they cry out (Caruth, 1996; Winnicott, 1974; Eshel, 2015, 2016, 2019a, b).

Clinical implications: working in total darkness

Eshel's theoretical innovations translate into specific clinical ways of thinking and working that address situations where the analyst must work, as Bion described, while "being totally in the dark." Her clinical material often illustrates experiences of being in states of massive dissociation, sleepiness, or extreme not-knowing, which for her has become closely connected with the most traumatic unknown and even the unknowable of catastrophic psychic trauma and breakdown. In a particularly striking case study (this volume), Eshel describes her experience of repeatedly falling asleep during sessions with a traumatized patient. Rather than seeing this as countertransference resistance, she came to understand it as a form of "projective realization" or "projective embodiment" of catastrophic psychic realities that had already happened to the patient. By allowing herself to be taken over by these dissociative states, allowing them to "be and become" her without understanding them but also without dread, Eshel creates a new therapeutic possibility. In Clari's treatment, the massive dissociation was transformed into "an attenuated, deferred dissociation" that could be held differently within the interconnected entity of patient-and-therapist—a massive yet sustained and tolerable experience. Through this process, the externalization of the dissociation within and through the analyst/therapist, and being within deep psyche-with-psyche connectedness, enabled the patient to dare approach, observe, and experience the dread of her inner self-other experiences.

The ethical dimension and faith

For Eshel, the willingness to surrender to this process reflects not just a technique but an ethical stance and an "act of faith" (in Bion's term). The analyst must have profound belief and trust in the psychoanalytic process, in the deep connectedness of patient and analyst, and in themselves as an analyst (2019a). This ethical dimension requires courage to stay and struggle within very difficult experiences, especially those that involve failure or lack of understanding. It requires a willingness to let oneself be touched and affected by the patient's suffering without retreating into theoretical defenses.

Compassion in therapeutic work: Eshel's unique expansion of Bion and Winnicott

An important yet often overlooked aspect of Eshel's theoretical innovation is her explicit integration of *compassion* into the very heart of psychoanalytic practice. While the concepts of empathy, containment, and holding are central to the works of Bion and Winnicott, neither explicitly developed a theory of compassion within their clinical frameworks. Eshel's focus on compassion (from the Latin *com*, "with," and *pati*, "to suffer"—literally, "to suffer with") represents a significant and radical expansion of their thought.

For Eshel (2013), compassion arises from the analyst's/therapist's willingness to be touched by the patient's suffering—to feel it within one's own heart and mind—and to remain *within* the experience without defensively retreating into theoretical understanding. This becomes especially crucial when working with traumatic states, where the patient's experience may be unrepresentable and cannot be approached through interpretation alone.

Why, then, did Bion and Winnicott not explicitly develop theories of compassion? Several factors may account for this omission:

1. **Historical context:** Both worked within a psychoanalytic culture that emphasized analytic neutrality and technical precision. Explicit discussions of compassion might have been dismissed as sentimentality or viewed as religiously inflected rather than clinically grounded.
2. **Implicit presence:** Although not named as such, elements of compassion are implicitly woven into their work—in Winnicott's notion of the holding environment and in Bion's containment and "passion" (*cf.* Eshel, 2019a, chapter 8).
3. **Theoretical language:** Both favored abstract, often deliberately ambiguous, theoretical idioms over directly emotional terminology.

Through this expansion, Eshel adds an essentially vital emotional and ethical dimension to psychoanalytic practice—one that complements and deepens the technical foundations laid by Bion and Winnicott. By bringing heart and compassion from the implicit background into explicit clinical focus, she restores to psychoanalysis the fundamental human connection that lies at the heart of therapeutic transformation.

Conclusion

Ofra Eshel—a fascinated–troubled analyst

As mentioned earlier, a *troubled analyst* is one who feels dissatisfied with the current state of psychoanalytic knowledge and seeks to create meaningful change that departs from existing traditions. What, then, troubled Ofra Eshel about Bion's and Winnicott's theories, leading her to develop her own distinctive contributions? To understand this, it is helpful first to consider how "troubled analysts" function within their respective theoretical communities.

Betty Joseph offers a good example. Working within the Kleinian tradition, Joseph became unsettled by the limitations of Klein's interpretive approach. She observed that interpreting past fantasies—the foundation of Kleinian practice—often failed to generate meaningful therapeutic progress. This clinical impasse prompted her to develop a new technique focusing on *here-and-now* interpretations of the transference relationship, which significantly advanced Kleinian theory while remaining within its framework.

Similarly, I believe Ofra Eshel's work grew out of specific clinical difficulties she encountered when applying Bion's and Winnicott's theories to more severely disturbed and traumatized patients. What troubled her was that their theoretical frameworks did not offer sufficient guidance for working with what she calls "the most unfathomable and unthinkable realm of traumatization that the psyche could not bear."

While both Bion and Winnicott recognized the centrality of the analyst's presence and the containing function, Eshel found that their concepts required further expansion to address the extreme clinical challenges presented by patients with unrepresented catastrophic psychic traumatization. The experiences of these patients could not be approached through traditional interpretation, or even Bion's notion of reverie and containment.

The specific gaps Eshel identified include:

1. **The need for an ontological rather than epistemological approach**: While Bion and Winnicott moved in this direction, especially in their later

works, Eshel was troubled by the predominantly knowledge-focused tradition in psychoanalysis. She strongly felt that for certain traumatic states, being-with the patient in their psychic reality is more crucial than knowing or interpreting.

2. **The need for explicit language regarding interconnectedness**: Though Bion spoke of becoming "O" and Winnicott discussed deep regressions, Eshel was concerned by the lack of a comprehensive framework to describe the range of needed states of patient-analyst oneness.
3. **The absence of a theory of compassion**: Neither Bion nor Winnicott explicitly developed concepts of compassion in their clinical frameworks, focusing instead on more abstract notions of containment and holding.
4. **Insufficient guidance for working with unthinkable and unrepresented traumatic states**: While both theorists acknowledged extreme psychological states, Eshel deepens their approaches regarding analytic work—especially in addressing what she calls "unrepressed unconscious," *level* **II**—the patient's radically unknown, unthinkable, unrepressed, and unrepresented traumatic psychic reality; experiences so catastrophic that they exist entirely outside of representation.

Cultural factors may have influenced these differences. As a Middle Eastern Israeli analyst rather than a British one, Eshel may have been less constrained by the British analytic tradition's emphasis on restraint and technical precision. Her cultural background may have enabled her greater freedom to embrace and articulate the emotional surrender and full engagement required for working with profoundly disturbed and unthinkable psychic realities.

However, the main driving force behind Eshel's innovations was not cultural but clinical—her determined commitment to reaching unreachable patients. Where Bion and Winnicott suggested possible directions, Eshel developed a comprehensive clinical framework for "being totally in the dark" with patients experiencing the most profound unthinkable and unrepresented psychic catastrophes.

By formulating concepts like the spectrum of analytic oneness, *Hinachechut* (presencing), the hearing heart, and compassion, she addressed what troubled her most: how to genuinely connect with and transform the deepest traumatic emotional realities, in particular the great unknown of mental catastrophe and early breakdown, that lie beyond representation, beyond interpretation, and even beyond more conventional ideas of analytic thinking, dreaming and containing.

References

Caruth, C. (1996). *Unclaimed Experience: Trauma, Narrative, and History*. Baltimore, MD & London: The Johns Hopkins University Press.

Eshel, O. (2009). To be "included" in the silence: On the silent patient and the analyst's "presencing." *Sihot—Dialogue, Israel Journal of Psychotherapy*, 23: 221–235.247.

Eshel, O. (2013). Patient–analyst "withness": On analytic "presencing," passion, and compassion in states of breakdown, despair, and deadness. *Psychoanalytic Quarterly*, 82: 925–963.

Eshel, O. (2015). The "hearing heart" and the "voice" of breakdown. In L. Aron & L. Henik (eds.), *Answering a Question with a Question: Contemporary Psychoanalysis and Jewish Thought, Vol. II: A Tradition of Inquiry* (pp. 133–152). Boston, MA: Academic Studies Press.

Eshel, O. (2016). The "voice" of breakdown: On facing the unbearable traumatic experience in psychoanalytic work. *Contemporary Psychoanalysis*, 52: 76–110.

Eshel, O. (2017). From extension to revolutionary change in clinical psychoanalysis: The radical influence of Bion and Winnicott. *Psychoanalytic Quarterly*, 86: 753–794.

Eshel, O. (2019a). *The Emergence of Analytic Oneness: Into the Heart of Psychoanalysis*. London: Routledge.

Eshel, O. (2019b). The vanished last scream: Winnicott and Bion. *Psychoanalytic Quarterly*, 88: 111–140.

Eshel, O. (2023). When deadness breaks in: Surviving, being-with and a moment of "at-one-ment" in analytic work within deadness and emptiness. *Modern Psychoanalysis*, 47: 145–171.

Freud, S. (1933). The question of a Weltanschauung. In J. Strachey (ed. & trans.), *The Standard Edition of the Complete Psychological Works of Sigmund Freud* (Vol. 22, pp. 158–182). London: Hogarth Press.

Govrin, A. (2015). *Conservative and Radical Perspectives on Psychoanalytic Knowledge: The Fascinated and the Disenchanted*. London: Routledge.

Pepper, S. C. (1942). *World Hypotheses: A Study in Evidence*. Berkeley: University of California Press.

Winnicott, D. W. (1945). Primitive emotional development. In *Through Paediatrics to Psychoanalysis* (pp. 145–156). London: Karnac, 1992.

Winnicott, D. W. (1974). Fear of breakdown. *International Review of Psycho-Analysis*, 1: 103–107.

Part II

The enigma of telepathic dreams

Chapter 4

Where are you, my beloved?

On absence, loss, and the enigma of telepathic dreams

Ofra Eshel

> It is a very remarkable thing that the *Ucs.* of one human being can react upon that of another, without passing through the *Cs.* This deserves closer investigation … but, descriptively speaking, the fact is incontestable.
>
> (Freud, 1915, p. 194)

> If only one accustoms oneself to the idea of telepathy, one can accomplish a great deal with it—for the time being, it is true, only in imagination … All this is still uncertain and full of unsolved riddles; but there is no reason to be frightened by it.
>
> (Freud, 1933, p. 55)

> It might be compatible with the idea that there is some mental phenomenon which is not bounded by what I can see and what I can hear, what I can smell and touch and feel … I suspect it is one of these things called 'extrasensory perception', but that it is probably too crude. As our intuition continues to develop we get nearer to situation where we seem to be aware that the boundaries of our mind are not our physical boundaries, not yet the boundaries which are imposed by our central nervous system. That is more like a guess, or a 'hunch', than anything one could call evidence or fact. But it may be a fact one day.
>
> (Bion, 1990; Rio de Janeiro - Two, 1974, p. 92)

> The analyst has to be able to tolerate ignorance – his own – and his being in the presence of a mystery, a half-truth. This seems to make it possible for the mind to have an experience in which it can grow.
>
> (Bion, 1990; Rio de Janeiro - Six, 1974, p. 131)

DOI: 10.4324/9781003674078-7

> So, touch with both ends at once, touch in the area where science and so-called technical objectivity are now taking hold of it instead of resisting it as they used to … touch in the area of our immediate apprehensions, our pathies, our receptions, our apprehensions because we are letting ourselves be approached without taking or comprehending anything and because we are afraid.
>
> (Derrida, 1988, p. 13)

Dream telepathy (especially patients' telepathic dreams) and related telepathic phenomena in the psychoanalytic context have been highly controversial, disturbing "foreign body " ever since telepathy was introduced into psychoanalysis by Freud in 1921.

In Laplanche and Pontalis's dictionary *The language of psychoanalysis*, there is no mention of telepathy or related phenomena in the psychoanalytic context. Yet, over the years, sporadic psychoanalytic writings on possibly telepathic experiences, and particularly patients' telepathic dreams, have accumulated and amounted to a body of clinical observations that deserve serious consideration. However, this was met with trepidation, from Freud's first article on this subject (written in 1921 but only published posthumously 20 years later) to Stoller's paper, 'Telepathic dreams?', written in 1973 but published posthumously 28 years later by Mayer (2001). Even this cursory information brings us directly and intriguingly into the heart of the controversy over and resistance to the idea of telepathy, which forced itself like "a foreign body" into psychoanalysis (Freud, 1933; Major & Miller, 1981; Torok, 1986; Derrida, 1988)—"a crypt that threw psychoanalysis, Freud included, into confusion ever since the 1920s" (Torok, 1986, p. 96). Indeed, a disturbing, "impossible" topic in "the impossible profession" (to use Freud's, 1937 locution). Delving into the profound mystery of telepathy in psychoanalysis is thought-provoking and complex, fraught with astonishment and discomfort often verging on a deeper trepidation (Eshel, 2006, 2019a, 2019b).

In the present chapter, I will focus and explore the profound enigma of patients' telepathic dreams from *my own analytic experiences* with them. But, to me, this is a crucial point. For it was only when I was faced in my practice with telepathic occurrences—unusual, surprising, rare, and inexplicable—that my interest in them and my search for an explanation evolved. There were five 'telepathic' dreams by five patients over my 35 years of clinical experience—dreams that 'knew' or occurred in the very place, time, and experiential state that I was in then. They made it absolutely necessary for me to presume the possibility of information transfer between patient and analyst in another, different way, one that goes beyond ordinary senses and speech. In this way I arrived at telepathy (from the Greek: *tele*—far, distant + *pathos*—suffering, intense feeling), a term coined by the English psychologist Frederic Myers in 1882 to "cover all cases of impression received at a distance without the normal operation of the recognized sense organs" (Royle, 1991).

This process evolved over time: The first two 'telepathic' dreams took me by surprise when my patients recounted them (several years apart), but I then pushed them to some remote corner of my mind. My approach changed only when such dreams recurred three more times over the years with other patients. These—starting from the third dream that I will present here in detail—remained in my thoughts, seeking to be resolved.

"Allow ourselves to be touched, wounded, and demolished in our own *being* … in order to try to approach what is radically other" (Pontalis, 2003, p. 11). I believe that, over time, I allowed my patients' telepathic dreams to touch and strike me. I let the feelings of incomprehension and discomfort invoked by these dreams linger in my thoughts, and I tried to psychoanalytically fathom their meaning, essence, and enigmatic emergence in the analytic process. It also led me to the intriguing psychoanalytic literature written over the years on the vicissitudes of the psychoanalytic encounter with telepathic dreams (Devereux, 1953; Eshel, 2006, 2019a).

I will now describe this third encounter with my patients' telepathic dreams and then the understanding that has crystallized in me over the years, which has found an echo and backing in the psychoanalytic literature.

Case illustration: "you alone knew how to wait/search"

Background

Effie (Efrat) came to analysis because of feeling increasingly unreal and detached from her husband, her four-year-old daughter, and her immediate environment, feelings unrelated to external circumstances. She would later add that these feelings had perhaps intensified since her daughter was about six months old.

At the beginning of the analysis, Effie recounted the dramatic story of her early childhood. Both her mother and maternal grandmother were Holocaust survivors. They had fled with a neighbor's family from their home in Poland to Russia. Her mother's husband of barely a year and her mother's father, along with the rest of the family, were due to join them a few days later but were caught and sent to concentration camps, where they perished.

During the war, Effie's mother and grandmother survived extreme hardship, hunger, and mortal terror. At the end of the war, they immigrated to Israel and attempted to rebuild their lives. Not a single relative, close or distant, had survived. Despite exhaustive efforts, they found no one who could provide additional information about what had happened to the rest of the family. They were totally alone; even the neighbor's family, with whom they had escaped, had immigrated to a different country.

Effie's mother found work and, a few years later, remarried and had two daughters, of whom Effie was the younger. During that period, with the help of her mother, who lived in close proximity, she stopped working and began studying at university.

Then, a crucial, devastating event occurred in their lives, an event about which Effie had only partial knowledge. When she was about ten months old, her mother's first husband suddenly reappeared. Effie did not know how he had found her mother, whether and how many times they had met, or whether they had only communicated by letters or phone. Apparently, they did meet. He too had remarried and had two young children, although Effie did not know who had remarried first; it seems they had remarried about the same time. He reappeared and then disappeared forever; Effie did not know whether he lived in some distant part of Israel or abroad. But he was never seen or heard from again. She did not know whether this had been a joint decision.

Effie's mother then withdrew and shut herself in her room. She would not respond, would not relate, and refused to see anybody. Her mother (Effie's grandmother) was called upon to help out and moved in with the family. She was a caring, devoted woman who mainly attended to meals and the family's other basic needs. Only two sounds cut through the silence in the house: the radio, which all day long and most of the night was tuned to the program *Searching for Lost Relatives*, and the song "Wait for me and I'll come back," which Effie's mother listened to over and over on the record player, alone in her closed room. Effie's father would return from work and sit on the balcony, sucking at his pipe in silence and staring out into the garden; at first, he slept in the living room, and later the balcony was enclosed so he could sleep there.

After about ten months, Effie's mother came out of her room and switched off the record player, and the song was no longer played. She went back to university, immersed herself in her studies, made up the year she had missed, continued studying and, in time, carved out an impressive academic career in her field. Effie's grandmother, replaced by a nanny, returned to her own home, but continued to be actively involved in their lives at home. The radio continued to broadcast *Searching for Lost Relatives*, but at a reduced volume, and only when Effie's mother or grandmother were home; they both continued to listen to it anxiously. Only once a year, every year, from the eve of Holocaust Remembrance Day to its end the following evening, would Effie's mother light a memorial candle and play the record once again in her room, and the sounds of the song "Wait for me and I'll come back," by now scratched and worn, would reverberate relentlessly throughout the house all that night and day. The candle burned, the song played, and Effie's mother remained shut in her room every year on that day. When Effie quoted me the words of this familiar old song, they suddenly seemed so harsh, poignant, and painful to me:

Wait for me, and I'll come back!

Wait for me and I'll come back!
Just you truly wait,
Wait when Autumn's dreary rains
Wait when snow is falling fast,
Wait when summer's hot,
Wait when yesterdays are past,
Others are forgot.
Wait though from that far-off place
No letters come to you.
Wait when others cease to wait,
All who waited too.
Wait for me and I'll come back!...
Even when my dearest ones

Say that I am lost
Even when my friends give up…
Wait, don't give up hope.

Wait for me and I'll come back,
Defying every death!
'What a bit of luck!' they'll say,
Those that did not wait.
They will never understand
How amidst the strife,
By your waiting for me, dear
You have saved my life.
How I made it, we shall know,
Only I and you.
You alone knew how to *search*
As no other knew.
(Konstantin Simonov, 1941)

"You alone knew how to *search* as no other knew," Effie recited the last line. "You alone knew how to *wait,*" I corrected the word, unable now to recall if silently or out loud, and not yet knowing that she had thus conveyed to me, without my understanding, the very heart of the telepathic occurrence.

Apparently, after that very difficult year, family life in Effie's home returned to normal. They talked little of feelings—"but maybe it was also like that before the crisis," said Effie. It was only years later, in late adolescence, that Effie learned from her sister and an elderly relative on her father's side about "the hard year." It began with the relative's comment that Holocaust Remembrance Day was so sad in their house, not just because their grandfather and the rest of the family had perished, but also because of "that man." Effie's efforts to find out more details were in vain; her sister and the elderly relative knew little. Her sister was four years older but had been only a young child at the time. Effie had never dared ask her mother and father, and they themselves never talked about it, while her grandmother refused to speak of those "old, sad matters." "My little girl" ["*Mein kind*," she would say in Yiddish], "we went through so many terrible things, you know, thank God, we got through it all, there's no point in talking about it, leave it alone, it's over and done with, everything is fine," she would say over and over, kindly but firmly, each time Effie broached the subject, and then fall silent or change the subject.

"Everything was fine" in Effie's life too. She did well in school, went on to university, married an older man and started a family; but the feeling of meaninglessness in her life grew ever stronger. Her grandmother died and then her father, and she "felt nothing." "I began to feel that my fate would be like that of Hannah in *My Michael* by the Israeli writer Amos Oz,"[1] she said. [The book tells of 30-year-old Hannah's growing withdrawal from her husband Michael and her young child, into a private, disconnected fantasy world, until her suicide]. Effie felt that the book's opening sentences very closely related to her: "I am writing this because people I loved have died. I am writing this because when I was a child I was full of the power of loving, and now that power of loving is dying. *I do not want to die*" (1972, p. 1, Effie's emphasis). And so, she came to analysis. She came to me because she had heard that my approach was Winnicottian.

The dream

During the first year of analysis (of four times a week, on the couch), Effie conveyed pervasive feelings of not belonging and heaviness and particularly had difficulty talking. "Basically, I never talked. I don't really know how to talk about feelings," she said. "I know how to organize, put all sorts of things in order and then … a vacuum." She felt "so heavy, not understood, not belonging, not connected to anybody. Once I had such a need to belong, but I got stuck somewhere in the middle." I felt her agonizing loneliness. She was very conscientious about coming to analysis, rarely missing a session or arriving late, but feared and blocked all feelings of connection, neediness, and dependence. In the sessions, I often felt that I had to hold her firmly lest she slip away through the empty spaces in her words. Yet, as the year drew to a close, a gradual, subtle shift seemed to occur in her tone of voice and in her intense feelings of isolation and desperateness.

The dream I describe was recounted at the beginning of the second year of analysis, on a Thursday, the third session of the week (we had no sessions on Wednesdays).

Effie began by saying she was "feeling better now." She was silent for a moment, then continued that she was "coming back" from being detached; she had had two difficult days, and everyone said she had been completely detached. She fell silent, then went on. Her husband talked to her but she couldn't hear. It seemed to her that I too had been detached on Tuesday, maybe also on Monday. She was silent again. I asked her, whether she thought that her being detached was related to my being detached. She said haltingly, "My body feels weightless. Floating. Not a pleasant feeling. Frightening." She was speaking with great difficulty. I said, "Effie, you were talking about my detachment and you became detached. Come back down to me and tell me what's happening." She slowly began to say that she had slept poorly the previous two nights, on Tuesday and Wednesday. Last night, she awoke very early and remembered a dream, which she then recounted (As is my habit, I wrote the dream down as she told it, and it is presented here verbatim).

> *What I remember is that I am in a different country, hurrying to the place where my father is buried, which I know is about to close at four o'clock. I manage to get there a few minutes before, go into some sort of entrance hall and from there I see that the gate I have to go through is closing. It's no longer possible to go in. I try to persuade the gatekeeper to let me in. I explain to him that I've come from a different place, far away, and I've already come in, and it's very important for me to come in because not being there, and he lets me in. And then I go into some sort of room, with a picture of my father hanging on the left, and next to it several other pictures. Like below the wall, underneath the floor, that is actually where my father is buried, it's not clear to me whether alone or with other people. I don't remember. It's as if the whole way he's buried is so different. And it's as if also in the dream I feel myself different. The entire time I'm someone else, I think. I'm not alone, I think.'*

She was silent and then continued,

> I usually don't manage to explain how important things are for me. I don't feel good about that. I feel myself not understood. That's how it feels to me—people don't understand me, then I become very tense, and then everything gets messed up. But here *I said, 'I've already come in. I've come from far away, it's very important for me to go in, let me come in', and he lets me in.*
>
> And my father's picture. A beautiful picture. He's smiling. There's a feeling of longing. That's something very new, this dream. Up to now my experience with dreams was that they confirm things I've already experienced in life, confirming them through a different medium.

I listened in astonishment to the dream and to the things she said. She dreamed the dream on Wednesday night, and Wednesday afternoon I had attended a memorial service in the cemetery for my own father, which began at 4 o'clock. And I had felt intense longing. I had been very attached to my father, and, around the time of the memorial service this year, due to certain family issues, I had especially missed him. I am certain that Effie had no way of knowing where I had been that day. I also realized that I had indeed been detached on the Tuesday, and perhaps also on the Monday, without being aware of it.

What encounter with me was Effie struggling for beyond the disconnection, beyond the closed gate, in spite of death and deadness? It was as if she had entered my mind, had been in a place and time I had been in, inside the longing I had felt. "I've come from a *different place, far away*, and I've already come in, and it's very important for me to come in because not being there," she had said to the gatekeeper, and he let her in. Who was it that was "not there"—her, me? The old deep scar of absence had suddenly reopened, speaking, pleading.

I deliberated whether to tell her all this; I asked questions about the dream and more was said, mostly about her parents, especially her father's years-long emotional distance from her world. Finally, about ten minutes before the end of the session, I decided to tell her, since so much had not been told to her in her life and had not been talked about with her. I said, "You know, Effie, yesterday I was really in the cemetery for my father's memorial service, at four in the afternoon. And maybe this affected my being detached and your being detached and your dream."

She remained silent until the end of the session and then said, "It is amazing and frightening how much things that happen to you affect me. Do you understand the enormousness of your responsibility?"

"Cry open in a forest of frost, in a dawn of cornflowers": the telepathic dream between absence and complete loss

> O my God, what am I
> That these late mouths should cry open
> In a forest of frost, in a dawn of cornflowers.
> (Sylvia Plath, 'Poppies in October,'
> 1962, *Ariel*)

In thirty-five years of clinical work, I have encountered five telepathic dreams. These five dreams were sporadic occurrences over the years. Yet they always appeared at emotionally charged, significant moments in *my* life and involved the precise details of time, place, sensory impressions, and experiential states that I was in at that time—dumbfounding *informational* details, not merely experiential-emotional details—that the patients could not have known through ordinary sensory perception and communication. All were connected to matters of life and death (in this order): a young female patient's dream in which *I was telling her that I was pregnant*, which she dreamed on the very day I found out that I was pregnant (with my eldest daughter); a dream of a male patient who "knew" I had miscarried (a different pregnancy five years later) when I canceled the sessions on those days; Effie's dream on the night of the memorial service for my father, which was where I was at—in place, hour, and emotional state—on the same day; a detailed cemetery dream by a male patient during the week that both my in-laws died within two days of each other; and a dream about a dying woman that a female patient dreamed three days before my mother's death—during a period when I would leave my mother's deathbed to carry on my analytic work—which depicted very specific details of the situation with my mother on those days, with dumbfounding precision.

All the telepathic elements were unique to these particular dreams and did not recur in these patients' other dreams (see also Stoller, in Mayer, 2001; Ullman, 2003). The first patient was in psychotherapy, and the other four in analysis; the latter dreams were equally divided between men and women.

The explanations of telepathic dreams during treatment in the psychoanalytic literature stem from factors related to the traumatic childhood circumstances of these patients, the ensuing non-verbal, archaic mode of communication heightened in critical, emotionally laden moments, and the analyst's role in provoking telepathic dreams. In my effort to unravel and understand these enigmatic, abstruse phenomena, a specific set of experiences took on primary importance, combining these three contributing factors:

Each of these patients, during *early childhood* (aged a few months to almost two years), had *a mother who was absent, mostly absent-within-absence*, that is, a mother physically present yet emotionally absent from her child's early life, often due to the absence of a significant figure in her own life. In my case examples, it was the absence of the husband-father (except for

Effie's special story)—one case due to sudden death, and the others due to a temporary but prolonged (over six months) absence of the husband-father. In most of the cases, the mother's experiences of absence and separation were intensified by an earlier absence of one or both of *her* parents (due to the Holocaust, lengthy separation, or death).

Thus, the silenced cry of this abrupt and critical early catastrophic trauma resides in a world of primal attachment, in a non-verbal or pre-verbal period, with an ensuing fixation on an archaic mode of communication.

Winnicott, in a memorable passage, describes the formation of annihilating x + y + z degree of the mother's deprivation:

> The feeling of the mother's existence lasts x minutes. If the mother is away more than x minutes, … the baby is distressed, but this distress is soon *mended* because the mother returns in x + y minutes. In x + y minutes the baby has not become altered. But in x + y + z minutes the baby has become *traumatized*. In x + y + z minutes the mother's return does not mend the baby's altered state. Trauma implies that the baby has experienced a break in life's continuity, so that primitive defences now become organized to defend against a repetition of 'unthinkable anxiety' or a return of the acute confusional state that belongs to disintegration of nascent ego structure.
>
> We must assume that the vast majority of babies never experience the x + y + z quantity of deprivation. This means that the majority of children do not carry around with them for life the knowledge from experience of having been mad. Madness here simply means a *break-up* of whatever may exist at the time of a *personal continuity of existence*. After 'recovery' from x + y + z deprivation the baby has to start again permanently deprived of the root which could provide *continuity with the personal beginning*.
>
> (Winnicott, 1971, pp. 114–115, italics in original)

I would say that the mother who is absent-within-absence creates the $x + y + z$ degree of deprivation/absence, or this is even a case of *double absence*—z^2—which is imprinted in the nascent self and in the baby's inchoate relating to others.

It is interesting that McLuhan expresses similar thoughts with regard to communication: "In any medium or structure there is a break boundary at which the system suddenly changes into another or passes some point of no return in its dynamic processes. … [here] the boundary break had been passed" (1994, pp. 38, 40).

Balint relates telepathic dreams to a patient "in a state of intense positive dependent transference, which however was not fully appreciated and understood by the analyst" (1955, p. 32). But I have found that these patients, because of their early traumatic history, defend themselves against strong and endangering feelings of dependence and becoming attached. Thus, in the treatment process, they struggle to block dependence, and will not allow themselves (and the analyst) to feel their deep regressive yearning for the analyst, except in a buried, hidden way. This abruptly changes when, within this intricate situation, the analyst suddenly becomes emotionally (and sometimes also physically) *absent* because his or her attention is significantly diverted to other matters, often to absence in the analyst's own world. Under such circumstances, the patient's dread of reliving the deeply annihilating traumatic absence, the breaking of personal continuity of existence, now bursts forth—never, never again to return to such devastating absence and abandonment, to that maddening, unbearable loss of the early mother.

The telepathic dream is created in *the gap between absence and annihilating loss*, between separation and all-out complete loss; it forms *a psychic search engine to seek and find the analyst in order to halt the process of abandonment and prevent a return and collapse into the depths of despair of the early catastrophic traumatization.*

Indeed, if tele-pathy is "suffering at a distance (Greek: *pathos* + *tele*)," the *suffering because of distance, suffering over distance*, achieves its critical potential here. The telepathic dream ushers us into the very heart of pathos—the suffering, the intense feeling; the patient's pathos, the analyst's pathos. For whose pathos is it? Whose dream? The dreaming patient clings to the analyst *beyond the boundaries of separateness, separation, time, space, and known processes of sensory perception* in a way that is hitherto not scientifically explicable, yet it occurs. The patient manages to enter the analyst's mind and the analyst's private affairs, experiences, absence—but not fully; that is, in a necessary, uncanny way, to telepathically perceive the most salient physical and emotionally charged details, which the ordinary senses fail to provide. Yet not fully.

"The gate … is closing. It's no longer possible to go in. I try to persuade the gatekeeper to let me in," said Effie in her dream. Only on re-reading these dream words lately did I realize with astonishment how similar they are to the deeply pleading words and the sense of critical urgency that imbues the final prayer of the Holy Day of Atonement [at-one-ment], the prayer which forms the emotional climax of the pleas that resonate throughout the day—"Open the gate for us at this time when the gate closes, for the day is fading away." (*Neilah* – The Closing of the Gate)

"I explain to him that I've come from a different place, far away, and I've already come in, and it is very important for me to come in because not being there. And the gatekeeper lets me in," Effie continued in her dream. On those particular days, she detached herself from her real world and reached me while I was in a different, emotionally laden, distant place. "And it's as if in the dream I feel myself different. The entire time I'm someone else, I think. I'm not alone, I think" [verbatim].

The biblical story of *Ruth's cleaving to Naomi* comes to mind to describe the powerful kind of connection embodied-encoded in the telepathic dream. "For wither thou goest, I will go; and where thou lodgest, I will lodge" (Ruth, 1:16). Under the shadow of great loss, Ruth "clave on to" Naomi, her mother-in-law, as she left Moab, adamantly following her, refusing any separation or separateness, detaching herself from her own world, crossing boundaries, allowing no room for any further loss.

It can be said that the telepathic dream actualizes the possibility of primary, unmediated patient-analyst interconnectedness or analytic oneness in the deepest sense, revealing its power and radical quality.

> Telepathy [is not] an actual transmission of sensory perceptions or of cognitive material from one person to another … We must assume that every telepathic incident involves the temporary fusion of two emotionally linked individuals into one functional unit, re-establishing for a fleeting moment the original mother-child unit as it existed at an early developmental stage.
>
> (Ehrenwald, 1960, p. 53, 1971)

At the same time, it still implies, in its very name and quality, the ultimately irreducible, irremediable distance between two people.

In the telepathic dream, the patient's reach exceeds his or her personal boundaries, turns into a paranormal mode of seeking and receiving information, and reaches-grips-holds onto the analyst—"a psychic prothesis, a stretched-out arm, which reaches out mystically towards that which is far off and cannot be approached in actuality by physical means" (Hitschmann, 1924, p. 438).

Thus, the telepathic dream breaks through the emotional absence and brings the analyst back to the patient, even when it does not make the analyst poignantly aware of his or her emotional absence and the patient's suffering, as Balint (1955) emphatically maintains. And, at its best, the telepathic dream creates *a moment of bare at-one-ness* of patient and analyst (at-one with the other and within oneself), while facing their intense and enigmatic inner interconnection that has now been exposed—thus creating a new observation, a new understanding, a *new possibility*.

Should the analyst—the only one who knows about the telepathic occurrence—tell the patient about it? Opinions are divided on such issues as clinical caution, the analyst's anonymity versus disclosure, and the authenticity of patient-analyst dialogue. Thus, Ehrenwald cautioned analysts not to tell patients until a later stage of analysis, when they would be capable of dealing with the burden of such involvement, while at that time Eisenbud (1946) maintained that, when analysts are careful, gentle, and wise in their handling of telepathic experiences, they can bring about most helpful and meaningful results. Considering these different approaches, Shainberg (1976) writes of his fear that his patient might be scared by the realization of the extent of his involvement with his analyst, and chose to avoid risk by not telling the patient. Conversely, Mayer (2001) is resolute about the importance of expanding the ability of patient and analyst alike to examine *all* aspects of what the patient knows about the analyst within the analytic intersubjective relationship, including anomalous telepathic knowledge. She sees this as important both in terms of the psychoanalytic situation and clinical psychoanalytic thinking.

Undoubtedly, this is a sensitive, daring, self-revealing moment, which, at times, is no less difficult and delicate for the analyst than it is for the patient. But I feel that it is a meaningful, authentic, and unique (intrapsychic and interpersonal) moment, which allows analyst and patient a different kind of exchange—groping and evolving—while facing their intense and enigmatic unconscious interconnection that has now been exposed. It is a powerful moment of connection that both comes to life and is deepened by this exchange. As Derrida writes so evocatively,

> You say 'It was me', with a gentle and terrible decision ... You say 'me' the unique addressee and everything starts between us. Starting out from nothing, from no history... (committing yourself to it even for eternity) ...you gather it together without reducing it, without harming

it, you let it live and everything starts between us, from you, and what you there give by receiving. Others would conclude: a letter thus finds its addressee, him or her. No, one cannot say of the addressee that s/he exists before the letter['s arrival].

(1988, p. 6)

In concluding, I find that this account did not take me into the domain of occultism, but rather into *the occult of psychoanalysis and the psychoanalytic process*. It ushered me into the heart of the unfathomable *depth, intensity, and mystery* of the human psyche and its struggle to survive traumatization and retraumatization, and particularly of patient-analyst unconscious quantum interconnectedness[2] in the psychoanalytic situation and its "impossible" extremes, defying space, time, and personal boundaries.

Notes

1 *My Michael* by Amos Oz tells of 30-year-old Hannah's growing withdrawal from her husband Michael and her young child into a private, disconnected fantasy world, until her eventual suicide.

2 I have called this process in its extreme singularity "quantum interconnectedness" (from physicist David Bohm's [1980] phrase "the quantum interconnectedness of distant systems"), in order to convey the profound implications of this quantum-like psychoanalytic quality of experience (Eshel, 2019a).

References

Balint, M. (1955). Notes on parapsychology and parapsychological healing. *International Journal of Psychoanalysis*, 36: 31–35.

Bion, W. R. (1990). *Brazilian Lectures: 1973 Sao Paulo 1974 Rio de Janeiro/Sao Paulo*. London and New York: Karnac.

Bohm, D. (1980). *Wholeness and the Implicate Order*. London: Routledge.

Derrida, J. (1988). Telepathy, Royle N, translator. *Oxford Literary Review*, 10: 3–41.

Devereux, G. (ed.) (1953). *Psychoanalysis and the Occult*. New York: International University Press.

Ehrenwald, J. (1960). Schizophrenia, neurotic compliance, and the psi hypothesis. *Psychoanalytic Review*, 47: 43–54.

Ehrenwald, J. (1971). Mother-child symbiosis: Cradle of ESP. *Psychoanalytic Review*, 58: 455–466.

Eisenbud, J. (1946). Telepathy and problems of psychoanalysis. *Psychoanalytic Quarterly*, 15: 32–87.

Eshel, O. (2006). Where are you, my beloved? *International Journal of Psychoanalysis*, 87: 1603–1627.

Eshel, O. (2019a). *The Emergence of Analytic Oneness: Into the Heart of Psychoanalysis.* London and New York: Routledge.
Eshel, O. (2019b) Would clinical psychoanalysis shy away from delving further into the unknown? On the mystery of telepathic dreams. *International Journal of Psychoanalysis*, 100: 608–610.
Freud, S. (1915). The unconscious. *SE*, 14: 159–216.
Freud, S. (1921 [1941]). Psycho-analysis and telepathy. *SE*, 18: 177–193.
Freud, S. (1933). Lecture XXX: Dreams and occultism. In: New introductory lectures on psychoanalysis, *SE*, 22: 31–56.
Freud, S. (1937). Analysis terminable and interminable. *SE*, 23: 216–253.
Hitschmann, E. (1924). Telepathy and psycho-analysis. *International Journal of Psychoanalysis*, 5: 425–439.
McLuhan, M. (1994) *Understanding Media: The Extensions of Man.* Cambridge, MA: MIT Press.
Major, R. & Miller, P. (1981). Empathy, antipathy and telepathy in the analytic process. *Psychoanalytic Inquiry*, 1: 449–470.
Mayer, E. L. (2001). On 'telepathic dreams?': An unpublished paper by Robert J. Stoller. *Journal of the American Psychoanalytic Association*, 49: 629–657.
Oz, A. (1972). *My Michael.* Trans. N. de Lange. London: Chatto & Windus.
Pontalis, J. B. (2003). *Windows.* Trans. A. Quinney. Lincoln & London: University of Nebraska Press.
Royle, N. (1991). *Telepathy and Literature: Essays on the Leading Mind.* Oxford: Blackwell.
Shainberg, D. (1976). Telepathy in psychoanalysis: An instance. *American Journal of Psychotherapy*, 30: 463–472.
Simonov K. (1941). Wait for me and I'll come back! *Pravda*, January, 1942, A. Shlonsky (Trans.), 1943.
Torok, M. (1986). Afterword: What is occult in occultism? Between Sigmund Freud and Sergei Pankeiev wolf man. In N. Abraham & M. Torok (eds.), N. Rand (trans.), *The Wolf Man's Magic Word: A Cryptonomy* (pp. 84–106). Minneapolis: University of Minnesota Press.
Ullman, M. (2003). Dream telepathy: Experimental and clinical findings. In N. Totton (ed.). *Psychoanalysis and the Paranormal: Lands of Darkness* (pp. 15–46). London: Karnac.
Winnicott, D. W. (1971). *Playing and Reality.* Harmondsworth: Penguin.

Chapter 5

"To approach what is radically other"

Ofra's Eshel's "Where are you, my beloved?"

Mary Tennes

On the morning of October 7, 2023, I sat down to begin writing this discussion of Ofra's paper (Eshel, 2024) for the IPTAR Conference on Telepathy at which we were originally presenting on telepathic experiences. I opened my computer and wrote a first paragraph in which I was appreciating the chance to speak about her compelling presentation. Through her gifts as a clinician, writer, and scholar, I said, Ofra has played a central role in opening and substantiating the exploration of telepathic and other uncanny phenomena within psychoanalysis. She locates these experiences within a revolutionary approach to analytic work in which, extending Winnicott's and Bion's most radical ideas, she emphasizes the profound quantum interconnectedness between patient and analyst (Eshel, 2019).

Suddenly, the news began to flash across my screen that Hamas had attacked Israel, and the horror and grief of what was happening began to unfold. Ofra was in Tel Aviv, her home. I wrote to her; she wrote back that she had been in a bomb shelter but had just emerged. The trauma, grief, shock, and dismay of the situation were overwhelming. I stopped writing. And, in the days following, I continued to struggle with what to write. The atrocities of these unprecedented attacks left me wordless. In the wake of this disastrous situation, our conference was postponed.

Clearly, my discussion had suddenly been altered by the mind-boggling intersection of beginning to write at the moment Ofra was suddenly and literally under siege. Rather than having the luxury of focusing only on Ofra's paper, I now had to address these colliding realities: an exploration of analytic moments of "oneness," as Ofra calls them, between patient and analyst side by side with the most horrific moments of disconnectedness and Othering between one people and another. How to hold together these seemingly impossible-to-integrate events? One might think that talking about

DOI: 10.4324/9781003674078-8

telepathic dreams between patient and analyst is a cloistered conversation in the face of a world in which people are being recklessly annihilated. In contrast, I see these profound moments within analytic work as urgently relevant to the question of how we contend with the collective catastrophes we are now facing. I will attempt, by the end of this discussion, to somehow make that link.

One place to begin is with the fact of being changed by experiences that unexpectedly present themselves to us. This discussion, over time, has required an ongoing adaptation to the circumstances that have arisen. As the disastrous situation in the Middle East and the responses to it became dramatically, tragically heightened, I felt the need to revise what I said several times. And even later, given all that continued to unfold, both there and here in our country, I continued to make changes.

The fact of being altered is also at the heart of a conversation about telepathic and uncanny experiences within psychoanalysis. Awe-inspiring clinical moments like the telepathic dream that Ofra describes challenge our everyday convictions about sensory reality and disrupt the familiar ground upon which we orient and stand. They are shocking, frightening, amazing—and so inevitably invite the analyst and the analysis itself to open to the unknown. Such openness is not easy.

In fact, the exploration of the telepathic has, throughout the history of psychoanalysis, been foreclosed with great force. Beginning with Freud, analysts who have experienced the startling, inexplicable quality of telepathic and other uncanny clinical moments have frequently hidden these experiences for fear of risking their professional reputations (Mayer & Stoller, 2001). Freud himself insisted that his early experiments with Ferenczi and Jung on "thought-transference" between patient and analyst be kept secret, for fear that their exposure would cause "the psychoanalytic house to explode" (Freud, 1925). When analysts in the decades after Freud have attempted to report such occurrences, they have most frequently been viewed through a denigrating, rejecting lens: as unscientific, defensive, naive, regressed, or even mad (Eshel, 2006, 2019). In a field that purports to be scientific, the need to turn away from experiences that challenge our existing paradigm is a striking statement about the threats they pose.

Of course it *can* be highly threatening to let go of the ground upon which we base our conceptualizations of ourselves and the world. Yet doing so is, in a sense, the premise and the power of a psychoanalytic approach: to work through our defenses against that which might unravel our known identifications. In particular, the unnerving reality that telepathic phenomena expose is one of incomprehensible interconnectedness, analogous to what physicists refer to as "quantum entanglement," a proven yet still unexplained phenomenon in which two particles mysteriously act as if they were one entity even if separated by great distances (Bass, 2001, p. 694; Dillow, 2016; Eshel, 2019). To truly open oneself to a telepathic dream in which self and other are somehow mysteriously, inexplicably connected is to open oneself to experiences that upend our known, collective assumptions about reality and selfhood. And the willingness to explore the reality of such astounding interconnectedness between human beings seems even more critical in the face of the blind and terrifying dehumanization that we are now witnessing globally.

Yet how do we not turn away from that which poses a threat to our established ways of knowing? Ofra offers herself as an example of both the inevitable hesitation and the necessary courage involved. She tells us that in response to the first two telepathic dreams that patients brought to her, she "pushed them to some remote corner of [her] mind" (Eshel, 2019, p. 119; this volume) and only later, when three more such dreams entered into her practice, did she allow herself to face the incomprehension and discomfort they evoked. She quotes Pontalis (2003, Chapter 4), who speaks of "'allow[ing]' ourselves to be touched, wounded, and demolished in our own being … in order to try to approach what is radically other" (Eshel, 2019, p. 120; this volume). In beginning with this focus, Ofra highlights the profound receptivity that such moments require. In order to be true to our analytic enterprise, we must allow ourselves to be affected, de-integrated, unraveled. Like a caterpillar who, entering into a transformative cocooning process, literally turns itself into liquid, we are challenged to surrender to the loss of known ways of understanding and being.

In taking up this challenge, Ofra describes the case of Effie, for whom the traumatic legacy of the Holocaust became a haunting presence. Part of what I find fascinating about Ofra's presentation of Effie's history are the words she both uses and doesn't use to describe the central events. Effie's mother and grandmother, she says, fled from Poland, but the mother's father and husband, along with the rest of the family, "were caught and sent to concentration camps, where they perished." These last words are definitive, as though the deaths have been confirmed. And yet, a few paragraphs later, we hear that when Effie was ten months old "her mother's first husband suddenly reappeared." In a way that must reproduce Effie's experience, there is no commentary or explanation about the discrepancy between the original certainty and the new reality that presents itself so that the supposedly dead husband's sudden arrival shocks and confuses, leaving the reader in a kind of gap, or limbo. Through this wording, the ex-husband seems to appear like a ghost out of nowhere.

On the one hand, Ofra's conscious or unconscious use of language mirrors and evokes the dissociative disjuncture of the traumatic, the breach that occurs in the face of the unbearable. Like an apparition caught in the gap between life and death, Effie herself feels "stuck somewhere in the middle." Ofra had to "hold her firmly, lest she slip away through the empty spaces in her words." Entering into a state of "at-one" with Effie, Ofra doesn't simply describe her patient but also, in her writing, recreates Effie's experience so that we as readers feel it as well.

And yet I also think this interesting absence of explanatory language speaks to the topic Ofra has taken up: the difficulty contending with that which, like a telepathic dream, defies understanding. A telepathic dream arrives like an apparition: unsettling, spooky, enigmatic, disrupting the known framework of things. It challenges us to be receptive to that which unravels our understanding. And that is what Ofra does, listening "in astonishment" to the dream details, which mirror her own experience, and not retreating from the inexplicable.

On a Wednesday—the day of the week that Ofra and Effie didn't meet—Effie dreamed of going at 4 o'clock to the cemetery where her father was buried. She saw a beautiful picture of him and experienced a new feeling of longing. That same Wednesday Ofra went at 4 o'clock to the cemetery where her own father was being memorialized; she had been especially missing him at this time and felt intense longing. The telepathic link between Effie and Ofra and between dream and reality is stunning. What is also remarkable is that the other details of the dream play out between Ofra and her patient as they are being shared between them. Effie tells Ofra she had been feeling detached the previous two days when they met, and she thought that Ofra had been detached as well, something Ofra realizes is true. In the dream Effie sees that the gate she must go through is closing, but she is able to persuade the gatekeeper to keep it open and let her in. Ofra, it seems, was a gate that was closing. In a beautifully skillful clinical exchange, she addresses Effie's ghostlike detachment—in response to her own detachment—encouraging her to "come back down to me and tell me what's happening." Then, as Effie describes the dream, Ofra allows herself to be profoundly affected and altered by what she hears, becoming the gatekeeper who lets the gate open again. Effie is not only presenting a dream; she and Ofra are living the dream together as it is being told.

Part of what is so astounding about telepathic dreams is that they expose not only a mysterious, uncanny interconnectedness between patient and analyst but also between states of dreaming and waking. When the dream world and the waking world seem to touch, our everyday orientation to reality is challenged. Our assumptions about the separateness of self and other and of internal and external worlds, as well as our established sense of time and space, are momentarily suspended.

Current scientific discoveries support such paradigm-altering revisions in our orientation. In a beautiful article exploring the parallels between the theories of Wilfred Bion and those of physicist David Bohm. Robert Godwin (1991) notes that one of the "bewildering abstrusities" of contemporary physics is that its equations describe realities "which literally [cannot] be pictured in the mind; for the first time in history, science [has] produced a model of the universe which [is] beyond our ability to comprehend" (Godwin, 1991, p. 627). Bohm himself suggests that in order to approach an accurate understanding of reality, our familiar ways of conceptualizing have to be suspended. Our normal categories of thought, he says, cannot do justice to that which we are attempting to grasp. In his words, "the dissolution of thinking ... is the highest priority the seeker for truth can undertake" to be replaced by what he calls "intelligence" (Godwin, 1991, p. 634). This movement is akin to Bion's idea that the analyst must, each session, suspend memory and desire in order to release saturated forms of thinking and to be present for the "new" patient arriving each hour. Tom Ogden suggests that if we actually grasp what Bion is asking of us, we should be "stunned" (Ogden, 2015, p. 291).

And indeed, Bohm proposes a stunning, mind-altering model of the universe that requires a relinquishment of our most fundamental assumptions. The perceived world of separate, fragmented entities, he says, is merely a surface manifestation of an underlying "fundamental realm of unbroken wholeness" (Godwin, 1991, p. 628) out of which the sensory world of individual identities emerges. The world of difference, as we perceive it, Bohm says, is more holographic than fixed and substantial; interconnectedness is the foundational reality.

Contemporary science, in fact, has leaped remarkably past its Newtonian origins so that, as Sean Carroll, a prominent physicist, says:

> Quantum mechanics ... is one of the most impressive intellectual accomplishments in the entire history of the human race ... because every idea ... violate(s) some cherished notion that we had really clung to. We had this paradigm handed down by Galileo and Newton and that was how physics was done ... and quantum mechanics comes along and changes all of the rules.
>
> (S. Carroll, personal communication, 2024)

Psychoanalysis is similarly challenged to let go of the Newtonian origins that framed Freud's model of the mind. Telepathic dreams disrupt us not only in a momentary and personal way within the analytic encounter; they also challenge certain cherished psychoanalytic convictions.

From that vantage point, I would like to take up a complexity in Ofra's paper. On the one hand, she emphasizes the inexplicable mystery she encountered in hearing her patients' telepathic dreams, and she herself makes links to mind-boggling scientific discoveries, referring to Bohm and to the "quantum interconnectedness" such dreams expose, "defying space, time, and personal boundaries." But then, in an interesting turn, she attempts to "unravel and understand these enigmatic, abstruse phenomena" by explaining their occurrence as an expression of an archaic mode of communication in patients whose parents were traumatically absent. In defending against a return to such devastating loss, she says, the patient creates a telepathic dream, a pre-verbal mode of functioning that, like a search engine, reaches out to find the analyst.

Although I would be hesitant to assume that *all* telepathic dreams arise in the context of traumatic early experience, I too had a patient with a history of unbearable maternal absence who brought an astounding telepathic dream to me, and when I let her know about the shocking links between her dream and my life, she burst into tears, saying, "We are so connected!" (Tennes, 2024). These uncanny moments clearly can function within the treatment to reveal a deep and startling bond between patient and analyst when a profound connection may be urgently necessary. I also think these dreams can often function, as they did with Ofra's patient, to disrupt and move the analyst past his or her own resistances and into new forms of awareness and relatedness. Furthermore, the link between the shattering effects of trauma and the receptivity to experiences that dislodge the cohesiveness of our everyday orientation to reality is a territory which could use further exploration.

At the same time, I would make a distinction between exploring the *function* of telepathic dreams within an analysis and attempting to *explain* the awe-inspiring, disruptive realities they present. The reason such experiences have been so sequestered for decades is because they disrupt the familiar ground of our psychoanalytic paradigm and ask us to bear the absence of a framework within which to encompass them. A familiar concept like "unconscious communication" does not explain *how* such phenomena occur any more than the terms "quantum entanglement" or "spooky action at a distance" explain the unanswered mystery of intertwined particles. Furthermore, equating uncanny, telepathic experiences with primitive forms of psychological functioning can move away from something more startling about them. In archaic, pre-verbal modes of communication, self and other lose their separateness as a certain merger or fusion is sought. Telepathic moments, however, are often characterized by a quality of paradox in which self and other both are and are not separate. When my patient, stunned, said, "We are so connected," she was awestruck by the fact that while being two distinct subjects, like two particles at a distance, we were nonetheless, somehow, in a profound, inexplicable alignment.

When a telepathic dream arises in a treatment, we are challenged to remain open to its disorienting effects. Ofra, in fact, has an exceptional gift for this kind of clinical presence. Her book, *The Emergence Of Analytic Oneness* (Eshel, 2019), provides numerous examples of her capacity to risk letting go of familiar, comfortable analytic positioning in order to enter into the primal disturbance her patients bring to her and, in so doing, to transform what could otherwise seem to be intractable difficulties. As her first paper here demonstrated, in allowing herself to fall asleep session after session in front of her patient, she was, as Charles Levin underscored, willing to "cross the internal Rubicon" to enter into territory for which there is no pre-conceptualized framework. In her work with Effie, she was similarly willing to bear the disruptive impact of her patient's shockingly telepathic dream, which somehow "knew" crucial, concrete details about Ofra's life and experience. This movement beyond the parameters of established psychoanalytic technique and beyond the constraints of one's own resistances is the movement Ofra's work encourages us to explore. In a broader way, psychoanalytic theory as a whole is being challenged by increasingly frequent analytic reports of telepathic experiences to move out of familiar conceptual ground and to surrender to the confusion, trepidation, and awe that such moments present.

To return to the beginning of my discussion, I see this capacity to move beyond the familiar and to open to what is "radically other" as centrally relevant to the highly disturbing developments of this moment in history. Our temptation, in the face of threat, is to retreat to the established parameters of our identities. Individually and collectively, we try to protect and reconstitute ourselves by moving into states of certainty. We reinforce what we think of as "self," and the other becomes a fixed and externalized Other. Yet what Ofra demonstrates, in what she calls "presencing" and "at-one-ment," is the willingness to inhabit a more liminal realm in which dream and waking, self and other, both are and are not distinct. This is also the realm of the telepathic and the uncanny, a realm of paradox, in which the willingness to remain suspended in the in-between leads toward new possibility.

How, then, might we attempt to bring this willingness to bear on the destructive breakdown of our contemporary world?

In describing the analyst's capacity to enter into an analytic process, Ofra, using a biblical phrase from King Solomon, refers to "the hearing heart" (Eshel, 2019, p. 11). As psychoanalysts, she says, we move into states of oneness with our patients by daring to open our hearts to "the heart-break which is at the centre of human existence" (2019, p. 13). Psychoanalytic listening, she suggests, comes from a heart willing to be altered, even shattered, by what it hears. Ofra herself demonstrates this willingness in a way that provides a profound and inspiring model for clinical work. She allows herself to be affected, changed, or, as Pontalis says, "touched, wounded and demolished in her [own] being." She gives herself to the analytic process, allowing herself to enter and know the patient's trauma, letting the process use her for purposes beyond her own understanding. Her work—on the cutting edge of psychoanalytic theory and technique—not only offers us possibilities for our work as analysts but also ushers us toward the territory that I think our global situation demands.

At this critical historical juncture, we might ask what it could mean for each of us, in our own unique way, to similarly give ourselves to the traumatized world, letting our hearts be shattered, attempting to discover the cutting edge of our own capacities, and risking the movement beyond our own resistances. I think of telepathic dreams less as extraordinary phenomena than as momentary windows that open, allowing us to see what we ordinarily do not see: a deep, abiding interconnectedness between us underlying the divisions we so readily perceive and create. The path of openness is not an easy one, but it does, in our work and in our world, seem essential.

References

Bass, A. (2001). It takes one to know one; or, Whose unconscious is it anyway? *Psychoanalytic Dialogues,* 11: 683–702.

Dillow, C. (2016, March 30). Quantum entanglement: Action at a distance. *Space.com*. https://www.space.com/31933-quantum-entanglement-action-at-a-distance.html

Eshel, O. (2006). Where are you, my beloved? *International Journal of Psychoanalysis,* 87: 1603–1627.

Eshel, O. (2019). *The Emergence of Analytic Oneness: Into the Heart of Psychoanalysis*. London and New York: Routledge.

Eshel, O. (2024). Where are you, my beloved: On absence, loss, and the enigma of telepathic dreams. Presented at IPTAR Conference on Telepathy, June 2024.

Freud, S. (1925). Letter from Sigmund Freud to Sándor Ferenczi, March 20, 1925. In E. Falzeder & E. Brabant (Eds.), *The Correspondence of Sigmund Freud and Sándor Ferenczi, Volume 3, 1920–1933* (pp. 209–210). Cambridge, MA: Harvard University Press.

Godwin, R. W. (1991). Wilfred Bion and David Bohm: Toward a quantum metapsychology. *Psychoanalysis and Contemporary Thought,* 14: 625–654.

Mayer, E. L. & Stoller, R. J. (2001). On "telepathic dreams?" An unpublished paper by Robert J. Stoller. *Journal of the American Psychoanalytic Association,* 49(2): 629–657.

Ogden, T. H. (2015). Intuiting the truth of what's happening: On Bion's "notes on memory and desire". *Psychoanalytic Quarterly,* 84: 285–306.

Pontalis, J. B. (2003). *Windows*. Trans. A. Quinney. Lincoln & London: University of Nebraska Press.

Tennes, M. (2024). Tell all the truth but tell it slant: Psychoanalysis and the uncanny. *Contemporary Psychoanalysis*, 1–21. https://doi.org/10.1080/00107530.2024.2428584

Part III

Reinventing psychoanalysis for severe perversion

Chapter 6

Calamities and secrets, the power of the fetish

Clinical case

Margaret Rubin

> Time Lived,
> Without Its Flow.
> Denise Riley

S lived a life of secrets that were both intoxicating and shaming. The inanimate objects that soothed and contained him in his neglected childhood were never outgrown. In adulthood, these morphed into an all-consuming fetish, keeping him immune to the passing of time.

His older brother told him the only thing he remembered from S's earliest years were his screams, the screams their mother never seemed to hear. S told me at the end of our last session that he always knew when I was coming to the gate to get him because he could hear my footsteps and counted them each time I came for him.[1] Did he count his mother's steps as she came toward his bedroom door, only to turn away from her grieving, angry, frightened little boy?

S managed to survive his traumatic, calamitous upbringing by using his mind as a substitute for mother's care (Winnicott, 1949; Corrigan & Gordon, 1995), sustaining a buttressing and binding self-sufficiency and self-regulation that maintained what we called his "universe of one"—his privileged psychic enclave for his "isolate self" (Williams, 2019), which kept his unbearable desires for human contact split off and unknown. In his early elementary school years, he constructed "the studio," a mental workspace inspired by TV and movies where he could play imaginary roles to get him through each day. Over time his mind held an endless, omnipotent catalogue of facts and characters that never failed him—if I do this, this will happen, as when so and so did this, that happened. Through sheer repetition, he cobbled together a pseudo-self hiding his conviction that he was a cipher, a simulacrum. "I am nothing," he would often say.

DOI: 10.4324/9781003674078-10

Everything S experienced was a reiteration of what was already known and experienced, leaving him in a state of hopelessness about anything ever changing (Seligman, 2016). All of this was enacted in his use of his fetish—a collection of steel male chastity belts specifically designed for his body, preserving an illusion that he was intact and safe from his tormentors. I hope to contribute to our understanding of the complex challenges of working with severely traumatized patients whose fetishism helps them bind the unbearable, keeping them locked in fixed and repetitive patterns of living in a world in which time doesn't pass—what Scarfone (2015) calls "the unpast."

Meeting S

Pre-pandemic

S had a prior treatment with a classical analyst and hoped to make more progress with a relational analyst. He was an imposing 58-year-old White Italian American. Grounding his presence was his sonorous voice that lent itself to gravitas—a boon, he thought, not only to his career in finance, but in delineating boundaries with co-workers. He sought another analysis because his wife found him emotionally unavailable even after his initial analysis. At the end of the first consultation, he mentioned he had a fetish but wasn't ready to talk about it. Referring to it as a distraction among many, he called himself a jack of all trades and a master of none, all part of his "symptomology" [sic]. It was 18 months until he revealed his fetish.

The smell of pine needles and neglect was S's first description of his familial environment. His father came from an impoverished family and spent his latency and adolescence in an orphanage, whereas his mother came from a wealthy blue-blood family, very much the princess bride, or so his father first thought. Absent of affect, S offered facts about his family, education, career, and marriage. During these early weeks of twice-weekly therapy, his childhood affect seemed to live in the landscape of his external environment. He would tear up when describing the ineffable beauty of the mountains surrounding the town where he grew up, which only he seemed to appreciate, and described himself as a loner and a transactional kind of guy. Since most social relationships were not transactional, he was often uncertain of the role he should play, seizing up with anxiety, unable to leave his house.

Toward the end of the second month of treatment, he had this dream:

> *I am working as an assistant in a medical lab, probably yours, in a beautifully designed building reminiscent of Louis Kahn's architecture. The doctor I am doing an experiment with has me manipulate a patient's irises, which had two different colors—blue and red. Your couch is blue and last week one of your eyes looked like it had a hemorrhage. When I pulled the iris open, moths flew out, and when I started to close the iris, the moths flew back in.*

S identified me as the doctor and had no idea who the patient was. Not himself, he thought. The patient seemed to be without a body, just a blank head with red and blue irises. His associations to the moths were memories. "Moths turn to dust when they die, and so do memories." The dream suggested to him that a new treatment was underway and was transactional—he was helping me do an experiment. When I asked about his associations to manipulating the irises, he had none (later when he referred to himself as a "weekend photographer," I associated the irises to the aperture on a camera).

After this dream, S continued to give me facts of his life, past and present. He loved tinkering, taking automobiles apart, then putting new or used parts back in and changing the lenses of his many cameras. As he was talking about his love of reassembling objects, he remembered a moment of surprising contact. He had taken a break from perusing a photography magazine and walked to the horse stables near his home. He stopped to watch a solitary horse grazing in the encircled field. The horse seemed to catch his gaze and walked over to the fence where S was standing. Spontaneously, he put his hand on the horse's head feeling the heat and sweat of the horse. It was a moment of deep intimacy and S began to weep. This was the first moment of palpable contact between us.

A calamitous upbringing

S was born a decade after his older brother. He was an afterthought and knew nothing about his mother's pregnancy and his birth. What he did know was that his mother was incapable of taking care of him. As a small child, he remembered his naked mother with her large breasts and "vagina hanging out" wandering through the upstairs hallway looking for her bath, smiling vacantly at him but never engaging him in any way. He described her as a zephyr—the breeze he could never touch. It fell to his brother and, on occasion, his father to change his diapers and return him to his crib to be left alone. He wondered if they were rough in handling him as he often felt uneasy around them. At a certain point his father decided to hire a nanny as his mother evaded any form of maternal care. This began the revolving door of nannies—his mother couldn't tolerate any of them. S showed me pictures of himself with the nannies but couldn't remember them. Later he told me he doesn't like looking at himself in pictures and mirrors and often finds himself unrecognizable.

The picture S painted of his infancy and toddlerhood was grim. He broke his toys and mostly put them back together. He figured out how to swaddle himself, and when a bit older tore up sheets to make the swaddling easier—his mother never noticed the torn sheets. A bodily memory of being stuck in his small room for hours at a time in his wet soiled diapers was enacted in his recurrent dream of being imprisoned at the bottom of a hollowed out well, unable to climb up its greasy walls. He called this his echo chamber, endlessly reverberating with the sounds of his screams.

In first grade, his mother gave him a small brown paper bag to take to school for "show and tell." When it was his turn, he pulled her lace slip out of the paper bag. He was aghast and when some kids started giggling, their teacher quickly took him outside the room. After this, the school asked his mother to come in. He never knew if she set the record straight.

And then he revealed more about his interactions with his mother. When he was around three, she put him in a metal harness to control his physical activity, as she convinced herself he was hyperactive. A lead was attached to the harness so she could walk him around their neighborhood like a dog. Despite this, he loved being put in the harness—these were the first touches of hers he remembered. He wished he knew where she tossed it, likely somewhere in the basement, he thought, where she put all her junk. Frequently he accompanied his scantily clad mother down the basement steps to watch her methodically clip discount coupons she never used, yearning for her attention.

It seemed he had no dependable attachments except for the neighbor down the street who would drive him home from school when his mother neglected to pick him up and always had food for him if he was hungry. His father was a figure he generally avoided who was either emotionally removed or intensely enraged about something—as when he shot bullets into the kitchen ceiling while S sat at the kitchen table. S remembers many occasions when he would hear his father raging at his mother at night and the next morning she would appear with blackened eyes. He casually mentioned his father and uncle had been sexually abused in the orphanage. When I asked how he knew that he said it was something he always knew just as he knew his father's favorite form of intercourse was anal sex, which he assumed he must have witnessed. Or had his brother told him? His parents' relationship was violent, and he never saw any softness or affection between them. This is why he became his mother's caretaker—often he felt like her parent. At times, he had the uncanny feeling they shared the same mind. He was uncertain if his thoughts were his own or if she had implanted them.

Toward the end of the first year of treatment, he had the following dream:

> *I was in an elevator with a bunch of people. I was the only one who gets out when we reach the top floor. The roof was a frozen landscape. Lifeless. Two nasty twin boys on the tennis courts playing hockey—not real boys. Aliens. When I get closer, I see they are malevolent. I run back to the elevator. When I get there, they are right behind me. Someone outside the elevator doesn't make it in. Something comes after that person—devours him like a chicken wing. I squeeze into the full elevator, but the nasty boys get in too. Then the lights go out and I start hearing crunching sounds. They were crunching the heads of the people in the elevator. Mine too? Or was it the crunching of my teeth on their heads that I heard?*

S had few associations to his nightmare. I asked about the nasty twin boys. Maybe boys from his father's time in the orphanage, he offered. I mentioned his feeling of confusion in the elevator—he didn't know who was doing what to whom. Whose mind was it? (I thought his dream had themes of disembodiment and undifferentiation). The nasty boys crunching the heads of the people in the elevator seemed emblematic of terrifying castration fears—the scene he described felt weirdly sexually assaultive—I told him the dream, to me, felt sexually assaulting and wondered what he felt. He said he thought that too. I felt this exchange revealed his need for omnipotence, as whenever I told him what I was thinking or offered an interpretation, his response was always "I already knew that." Before this dream, he had mentioned that his mother wouldn't let him join the cub scouts—they were a bunch of ruffians, "scruffy, nasty boys." I asked if the nasty boys might be a reference to his mother's description of the cub scouts. S said he never told me that and joked I was gaslighting him. (I was caught in his dissociative moment and said very little, as trusting his own mind was his primary survival mechanism.)

This dream seemed to open an area where danger and safety, and sexuality and castration, were distorted and constricted. He disclosed his fascination with restraints—he first tied himself up with a jump rope when he was six and found it more effective in feeling safe and contained than swaddling. This became ritualized in early adolescence when he felt he couldn't mediate his anger and was likely overwhelmed by his sexual desires. He lost his virginity at 16, liked girls and had several good sexual relationships in high school, joking that was the only thing normal about him. When I asked what he meant by normal, he explained that's what teenagers are supposed to do and that he learned what boys do with girls from watching TV and movies. Then, he mapped it out in the studio before trying anything.

His relationship with his mother became strained when he had his first girlfriend. Once after spending the day with her, he became enraged when his mother demanded he mow the front lawn. He screamed and ran upstairs to his bedroom to bind himself. Getting naked and bound up calmed him down, helping him regain control of his rage (and sexual excitement, too, I wondered). Without bravado he said this was the only time in his life that he experienced murderous rage, which terrified him. His mother found him in his bedroom closet like this. Horrified and angry, she screamed, "This shall not be allowed." Filled with revulsion for her, he remained frozen in the closet.

S became agitated telling me this and went on.

> My father would pee on iconic buildings and stole a painting from the prep school I attended when he picked me up after a onetime summer semester. That was his way of shitting on my experience. At least he went to work and lived in the real world.

S then told me his father had raped his older brother before he was born and that both his father and brother had "huge" penises, whereas his was "small." So much sexuality and rage were unleashed in his family, with hardly any safety and containment except what he provided for himself. I tried to remain a witness with my hand gently on his shoulder, helping him feel enough in control that my being a resilient background figure would eventually enable him to wander out into a more related field of our creation.

The fetish

The following week S began the first session by asking me if I knew what a male chastity belt was. I didn't. He then proceeded to educate me on the designs of these highly effective belts that restricted erections and delayed orgasm. I asked how many belts he owned. "Over 200." He had several storage lockers, and PO addresses where new belts could be shipped, as his wife was unaware of his fetish. At the end of that session, I asked if he could bring in a few belts so I could see what they looked like.

The next day he brought in a satchel filled with belts he kept locked away in his home office. As he carefully, and lovingly I thought, laid the 16 belts on my office rug, he described each one to me in detail, where they were made and the artisans who made them. His favorite belts felt like a second skin—all were custom-made. I found them aesthetically beautiful and told him if he hung one on a gallery wall, it would look like a Marcel Duchamp. S laughed and said I would have had a very different impression of his first chastity belt, which he had made from a broken old bicycle chain that he, much to his surprise, orgasmed in at age 11. And there it was right before our eyes. He had let the moths out of his irises, and they were not going back in. We both understood that his experience of being imprisoned in his crib, swaddling himself, wearing the harness, and tying himself up had been deeply inscribed in his body. The fetish provided him containment and safety, as well as the painful frustration, tension, and over stimulation that marked his infancy. Over time it became an entrenched part of his self-regulatory system. He felt in control of the affective swirl around him as he was untouchable whenever he wore the belt—his salve from his disastrously chaotic and destructive parents.

We agreed the following week to add a third session. He wondered if he would be using the couch as he disliked it in his first analysis—it was reminiscent of his echo chamber. I suggested eye contact was preferable for now. He looked directly at me saying, "I'd like to give this fetish up, but I don't know how to stop. 'This shall not be allowed.' Whose voice is that? I don't know how to do this, give this up." He looked disconsolate but didn't circle back to this until much later.

After this, he told me in detail about the pornography he looked at every morning before masturbating and making coffee—the pornography was all about restraints, men and women in restraints, and sex slaves in medieval torture devices. He especially liked imagining himself as a damsel in distress. Although he felt no sexual desire for either sex, it was exciting to imagine himself in their restraints—especially a strait jacket. His father kept a stash of Playboy and Hustler magazines in his bathroom, and he liked sneaking in there to look at them. S never felt aroused—the vaginas were unsavory, but he loved that the Playboy bunnies' outfits were constricting and uncomfortable. Even as a kid he knew his arousal was baked into the feeling of being in restraints. I asked if he was ever aroused when hearing his parents fighting, or when he saw his mother's blackened eyes. He hadn't but told me at times he "ratted" his mother out to his father knowing it would bring on a beating—like the time his mother drowned his two kittens their neighbor had given him. She didn't like cats or the neighbor. When he saw the drowned kittens, he called his father at his office. That evening he heard his father raging at her, and the next morning she had two bruised eyes. (Did the blue and red irises in his first dream represent his mother's bruised eyes? S experienced his mother as unleashed and "out there," whereas he felt his father's rage was overblown for effect. He was traumatically overexposed to the oversaturating sexuality and bizarre behaviors of both his mother and father and called their relationship a folie a deux.)

My understanding of S's dynamics deepened around this time. His mother's manic sexual behaviors and splintered thinking dominated his childhood. I wondered about his merger with her madness when he revealed the time he lost control of himself after moving to the West Coast. He rented a studio apartment and, upon realizing he had lost his keys, flew into a frenzied rage and broke the front door down with his fists and a tire iron from his car. The intense fear and rage he felt when locked out of his chastity belts suggested his fetish was a bastion against his mother's psychosis. (I wondered if he would have gone mad, ending up in a straitjacket, if he hadn't seized upon the chastity belt.)

The pandemic

Zoom sessions

Without the pandemic, I wouldn't have seen his home office. "Souvenirs" from his life fill every inch of the room, which is jampacked with four functioning computers on two large desks covered with magazines, piles of papers, pens, pencils and erasers. Floor to ceiling bookcases fill the walls with his vast collection of slinkies adorning the shelves. I am witnessing the workspace of a life lived without witnesses in his metaphoric basement, joining the ghost of his mother. I learn about the souvenirs, mostly trinkets purchased in airports that prove his existence in time and place. This is his shameless version of show and tell.

He tells me he doesn't know the difference between a keepsake and "stuff". Then shows me a stack of boarding passes that concretize his footprints from the year he flew to a different city every week for his job. He wonders if I would help him sift through his stuff once the pandemic is over—he wants to get rid of things but is afraid without them his memories will turn to dust. I tell him his things are stored in my memory and won't be forgotten, and when the pandemic is over, he can bring them to my office for us to sift through.

Seeing me from his universe of one has a salubrious effect on him. He speaks more freely about his anxieties. Whenever he wears one of his belts, he always puts on a pair of lacy panties over his belt, like the kind his mother wore, and then two women's bathing suit bottoms and a pair of his boxer shorts. (His ritualized attire is consonant with Celenza's hypothesis (2014) that wearing female garments embodies the desire to have it both ways, i.e., being a woman while remaining male.) I ask if he ever put on his mother's panties when he was a kid. He laughs, saying at age eight he swiped some of her lace panties and liked wearing them—they were soft and comfy. But the best part was feeling he was getting away with something. Despite knowing she couldn't keep track of anything, he was disappointed she never noticed. Nevertheless, he hoped she'd realize her favorite panties were missing, and he'd have the pleasure of making her feel crazy. When he bought his first chastity belt, he had the idea to wear women's panties and bathing suit bottoms over the belt and discovered that wearing them not only disguised the belt but also flattened his stomach. An unexpected plus, he joked. (Getting away with something was his primary identification with mother—on occasion he wore the belt to business meetings and sports events but stopped during the pandemic and never risked doing it again.)

His chastity belt was the manifestation of all his neglect, abandonment, terror, and self-soothing, along with the harness that became eroticized when his mother put him in it. We examine his conflicting emotional states around their sadomasochistic relationship, e.g., forgiving her and derogating her, loving her and hating her—a simulacrum of hatred and merger. Who is the doer and who is the done to? He plays both parts. His mother's message, or perhaps his own, "this shall not be allowed" is inscribed in the belt. He can't be castrated. The belt is his protective membrane from his tormentors. His pleasure is solely about his own excitement, which is his capacity to sustain his tumescence and delay orgasm for four to six hours. He is omnipotent, turning trauma into triumph.

This is a generative phase of treatment. The following dream suggested he was allowing himself to depend on me.

> *I was nodding off in your office. You disappeared into your home and returned with an old, checkered oilcloth that had been on my mother's table in the basement and wrapped me up in it. I must have been a child because you gently laid me down on your rug to sleep. When the session was over, you woke me up and walked me out to your back gate. And there was Bill Gates waiting to come in.*

"Why Bill Gates?" I asked. He reminded me to give him my invoice, or bill, at the end of every month and hand it to him as I walk him to the back gate. "Everything comes with a cost," he laments.

S felt he had never been attended to. Nonetheless, his dream about my wrapping him in the oilcloth and gently laying him on my rug suggested our relationship offered him a center of safety and containment.

> I needed to find a center and still do whenever I'm thrown off by something. I first started working on this in the studio and created a whole version of my lived personal nightmare that could be worked with at arm's length, entirely with data. My tool kit is my anger, which I can quickly turn into rage to annihilate the disruptor. I used to think of the monster within as a necessary defense against father, but he's just a blowhard. It's my defense against mother. I always suspected she was the one who assaulted my brother with her sadistic insistence on giving him enemas, which he hated. She's the monster I can't stay mad at—yet I still give her a free pass. I see her as I did then, wandering the upstairs hallway naked with her huge breasts and vagina hanging out. I feel her skeletal system living inside me. I've moved past her crimes and have forgiven her. Is this bizarre self-esteem?

Post pandemic

The inevitable enactment

Once back in person, S brings in a trash bag and two duffel bags filled with stuff for us to sort through and assembles them into two piles on my rug—what he should toss and what he's ambivalent about. We sort things out once he realizes his receipts and to-do lists have no emotional pull. The other stuff is nostalgic old clothes of his father's that never fit him but represent his veneer—he dressed like a gentleman. After deliberating, he ruefully decides to donate his father's clothing. Somewhat awkwardly, he shows me a large folder full of envelopes I had given him that no longer contain my invoices. This, he says, is a keepsake. Without fanfare, we discard his piles of receipts and lists in my garbage bin in the alleyway. As he walks the short distance to his car, I see his large folder clutched to his chest while holding the trash bag in one hand and the empty duffel bags in the other. His solitariness is heartbreaking.

After this he tells me he lives outside of time. What does being present look like? he wonders. The inescapable persistence of the past holds him hostage.

> My belts lead me to my body, which is always in dissonance, my baseline of aliveness. Eros merged with aggression. I am the architect of all the tumult. My merger with mother. All this lives within the configuration of the belt. What can possibly replace my obsession?

Despite this, he tells me he c is it possible? Being without it terrifies him. After some thought, I propose an addiction model might help him give it up for a time. How long, he wonders. I suggest we decide this once we see what feelings arise when he isn't using the belt, as it is the fetish that keeps him irretrievably stuck in the endless repetitions of his past. He nods anxiously but worries he won't know what to do with himself without his belts.

He remembers a dream fragment—he and his naked mother are entangled in a medieval restraint, a horrifying image forever linking them in his unconscious. Yet in this session, he brings in a piece of steel from an old belt that he is considering soldering onto another belt to make the restraint more punishing. And then I learn about the bots—the AIs that determine the length of time he stays locked in the belt. His goal is 20 to 24 hours, which he sometimes meets. The more at risk he is, the more excitement he has.

The longer the restriction, the more potent the orgasm once he is out of the belt. He explains the bots don't have control over the time—it's all an illusion. He can always get out. The universe of one prevails.

I feel I am tracking him well during this time. He tells me about his mother going berserk when he had a meltdown at age five. She knocked him over and sat on him, then flipped herself over, lying on top of him, breathing into his face. He found her open mouth and breath disgusting. Feeling her genital area on his felt horrifying. Nothing further happened, but he couldn't make sense of it. "Maybe that's when I first became her caretaker—she was a barnacle. I couldn't make her well and took her crazy impairments as my own."

He has a spate of dreams about being a woman and wonders if the people in his dreams recognize this. In one dream he is in a sanctuary sitting on a toilet "doing his business" when he realizes he has no genitals. Two deacons are nearby, watching him. One of the deacons starts to undress and when he sees his large breasts realizes the deacon is a she, and the she is his mother. He often feels genderless in the belt and was wearing the belt when he had this dream. Theorizing that the male and female parts of his psyche were corroded by his parents, he thinks he is in a "self-correction" phase with me. A few weeks later he has the first sex dream he's had in decades. He and Elizabeth Holmes, the jailed Theranos founder, are having passionate sexual intercourse, and he wakes up with an erection and quickly goes into the bathroom to masturbate. I ask if the dream suggests when he experiences his masculine and feminine parts in a 'self-corrected way,' he is more likely to feel sexual desire for a woman. He disagrees vehemently. "The vagina is horrifying and nauseating to me. You don't get it! Penetration feels like putting my finger in cookie dough" (I remember him saying early in treatment that contact with his mother was like putting his finger in cookie dough. "There was nothing there." I remain silent, thinking his depiction of the vagina as grotesque and disgusting reflects his earliest experience of his mother, as is his finger being in cookie dough. I consider that being genderless in the belt in his dream states protects him from his mother's unsavory sexuality. Is this what I missed? Or did my comment suggest I was endorsing his desire to have sexual intercourse with a woman? To get on with it? I wonder if sexual intercourse with a woman is unconsciously experienced as an infidelity to mother. Had she hoped her second child would be a girl—her clone, not a 'scruffy, nasty boy'? Was this what being female in his dreams suggest? Was his castrated self his penultimate gift to her?)

S seemed constantly annoyed with me after this and was using the belt incessantly. I found his obsessive need to understand every nuance of the belt exhausting but wasn't sure what was going on between us and how I had contributed to our stalemate. Had I sullied his relationship with the belt when I mentioned the word addiction? He had an expression on his face I hadn't seen before. A sneer?

> You don't understand the nuances of my experience in the belt. It's a metaphor for my survival. I am untouchable. Get it? I only reside in my body when I am in the belt. The noise in my head goes away when I wear it.

I ask about the noise.

> Father's critiques, mother's nothingness. Skin on skin makes me cringe. But skin on metal is erotic. You can't possibly understand me. You are from Buffalo. (Where did he get that idea?) You have had such a lucky life. You don't know what you are talking about half the time. You invite my rage.

I say, "Unwittingly I probably do contribute to your rage. But I'm not sure what's causing your anger now."

"When I was using the belt every day, you called it an addiction and said we should think of it that way. You had made an interdiction!" he said furiously. I remember, I say, and don't contradict him.

> I've been angry with you for calling my belt an addiction, which I know it is. I'm not stupid! But what you don't understand is the belt is my way of surviving my parents' relationship with each other and with me. Giving up the belt must come from me. My self agency! It has nothing to do with you! What you think means nothing to me!

After a beat, I say "I understand. Of course, it's your self agency. I'm sorry." I don't say I suspect our enactment is a reiteration of the fixed and routinized way he uses his fetish (Celenza, p. 128). Nor do I say that our enactment is about his conflict with me now that our relationship is in the transference. I believe his increased use of the chastity belt reenacted the time his mother demanded he mow the lawn and he refused to submit—my suggestion had pitted his will against mine, which he heard as a demand for submission rather than a surrender to the analytic process and held onto his reins even tighter. (I first wrote reigns, an interesting slip as I resisted his control.) When his rage finally erupted, he needed my recognition that I had threatened him. S apologized later for getting angry with me, worried I might be upset with him. I assured him I wasn't—there was no price to pay.

The break

After this I did my best to stay in his rhythm and ride out the lingering storm. Then a few weeks later as planned, S and his wife went away for a week. When he returned, I was on vacation for a week, which he had known about. After the Labor Day weekend, he texted me saying he and his wife were doing another trip and he'd be back by the end of September. He didn't return until the second week of October—he was gone six weeks.

The first session back, I told him how glad I was to see him. He smiled and told me about his trips. He said nothing about the break. I followed his lead. He talked about work and getting more fit, all very matter of fact.

And then he had the following dream later that week:

> *I'm playing poker with friends from college, and I am suddenly aware of my body. I could feel my musculature separate from my skeletal system. Very weird feeling. But with this division, I was seeing more. There was an arsenal of people around me. Parts of myself? Roles I've played? I keep them in an arsenal to be opened when I need them. Then I see all these ghosts walking through the room and I wake up.*

(I view this dream as a representation of reembodiment. His life, i.e., his musculature, is separating from death, her bones—all in the presence of his ancestors).

When I ask him what he thinks about the dream, he says,

> I think I need to stop using the belt. It's my mother's skeletal system, after all. How long do I need to keep carrying it? Did I tell you she was once apprehended by the police for hitting someone in a bank who told her she couldn't use their copying machine? And when I was a teenager, I asked her why she hadn't breastfed my brother and me. Cupping her

> large breasts, she taunted me saying 'I was saving these for your father.' I realize more and more how disturbed she was and how I absorbed it all. I think I am free to be myself, finally. Whatever that means.

He wondered when he came back if I thought he was going to quit analysis. I told him I felt that was a possibility but hoped otherwise. He tells me he had to take the break—he despised that word addiction, but knew it was true. If he was going to get better, the belt must go.

Three months after returning to treatment he has this dream:

> *I was the sole survivor of a disastrous plane crash and was wandering around this huge debris field in high heels, littered in body parts and airplane parts. I am pretty sure I am a woman. You were the tv journalist interviewing me. I wondered if you knew I was a woman. I didn't remember the crash and didn't want to talk anymore. I was exhausted from screaming and wanted to go home but didn't know where that was. You said let's find you a place to sleep and rest.*

As I focused on the dream images, he said haltingly, "This is not a typical dream for me. I know I am having a lot of dreams of being a woman. But you wanting to take care of me deeply affected me. You heard my cries." His screams were finally heard. In his dream, S was able to begin to experience the catastrophe of his childhood that until now had been unthinkable.[2] He had survived, but at such a cost.

Toward the end of December, he has gotten rid of all the French lacy underwear but is keeping some of the women's bathing suit bottoms. He is sick of the madness that pervaded his family and feels he was cut off in his own deadness, and despised himself. He remembers the time before meeting his wife when he stuck dildoes up his anus and fantasized about mutilating his penis.

> Every time I'd use the dildos, I'd hear a voice in my head saying 'Nasty, bad boy.' Why was I doing this? What was I punishing myself for? I think I am learning to reconnect to the suffering and pain I suffered alone. I think I am experiencing it now with you, and its different.

He quietly cries—his silence enveloping both of us. (S told me months before that he thinks his mother called him a "nasty bad boy" when he was a kid. When he repeated these words, I assumed it was his mother's voice. S hearing it as 'a voice in his head' suggested their merger was seamless when he wore the chastity belt fantasizing about mutilating his penis.)

Tinkering is now seen as his primary organizing principle, not anger. It began with the toys he first took apart, the sheets he tore up, the jump rope he used to bind himself, the broken bicycle chain that he fashioned into a belt, and later the lenses, automobile and belt parts he loved swapping out. All this compensated for the profound loneliness and dissonant sexual and aggressive feelings that permeated his life in his childhood room. The problem with the belt, he tells me, is that it thwarts his independence, keeping him frozen in a deadened space. "I am forever sharing my mother's mind. What happened to me? Do you think I was sexually abused? Assaulted like my brother? Am I doing penance? But for what?" I tell him we may never know, but we do know that his psyche was continually appropriated by his mother. Their merger lives on in the frozen deadened space. S says, "Uh-huh … interesting … I never thought of that."

Soon after this, he became more engaged when talking about the company he worked for and the colleagues he liked. He casually mentioned his work was more enlivening since he had stopped using the belt. I thought I had misheard. I hadn't. I told him he was holding out on me. He laughed and said, "You are the last to know, but since you are the only one who knows, that ain't so bad." He had stopped using the belt seven weeks before.

Much to his surprise and mine, he is less anxious without the belt. He feels more present and no longer engages in repetitive tasks to lose time.

> I feel more aliveness in my body, more me. I'm doing photography again, and its good! Spooning my wife is different—I feel myself spooning her. After our long drought, I think I may want to have intercourse again. For the first time, I am hopeful my life will continue getting better. And I am spending less time looking at my bondage sites—though I still fantasize about restraints.

As an afterthought, he tells me he was contacted by one of the German belt makers about a new belt. He wanted to have one made but knew he wouldn't and deleted it from his email. He asks if we can add a fourth session, which we do.

He feels the chastity belt obstructed his relational aliveness. In these months without the belt, he feels lighter, less encumbered, and less drawn to the past. He calls this the honeymoon phase but worries it won't be sustainable, as the mesmerizing sounds of the Sirens live in the chaos and terror of his dangerous pathological family. This is the seductive lure of his chastity belt. Once he locks himself in, his triumph is assured, as, like Odysseus, he remains restrained, defeating his tormentors.

The addition of the fourth session comes at the right time. He is rewatching Andrei Tarkovsky's film The Mirror. He relates to the unconscious of the dreamer—she, like he, lives in the collapse of time where the past is inescapable. And then he associates it with Shakespeare's Titus Andronicus. He recounts the plot:

> Titus's daughter has her tongue cut out and hands chopped off by nasty twin boys. He finds his maimed daughter and encourages her to spell out her attackers' names with her feet. Titus murders the nasty boys and boils their bodies in their own blood. He seeks retribution by making pies out of their heads and feeds them to their depraved mother.

I am surprised by his association with Titus Andronicus.[3] Was Shakespeare's unmediated violence nostalgic? But he had repressed one critical fact. Titus Andronicus' daughter was first raped by the two brothers, and later disfigured. I remained quiet, wondering if the daughter's disfigurement reflects his exhaustive on-going oscillation of identification and disidentification with his mother's body and psyche. I don't mention the nasty twin boys but am intrigued he is bringing them up again—Shakespeare did not refer to the warrior brothers as "nasty twin boys." Whom do they represent? So many permutations come to mind as the members of his family are undifferentiated pairs living in mayhem under one roof. I am struck by an image of the nasty twin boys as himself without genitals and his mother dressed as a deacon. He then says, "I am maimed like the daughter. That's who I am. Disfigured" (Just like the other nasty boy, I think). He begins to weep.

I feel I understand S's experience with his seductive manic mother. Where did her body boundaries end and his begin? Early on he told me he felt his mother's intentions toward him were untoward. From the very beginning, S's story was about his mother's vagina and the trauma and shock of castration by a mother who disallowed any autonomy. He found the vagina "horrifying and nauseating" and referred to her vagina "hanging out," which likely reflected his confusion with the suspended male genitalia. Her naked body, notably her exposed vagina, was the medium for all her communications. All of this was exacerbated by his parents' hyperreal sexual and psychotic relationship that kept him lost and abandoned. Because S's mother was incapable of providing a place of imaginative freedom and play, she couldn't provide disillusionment, resulting in delusion replacing disillusionment, which contributed to the creation and use of his fetish. She had repeatedly traumatized him by her unrelenting nakedness that expropriated his mind and body. By carrying her skeletal system, S could not escape her—their "nasty twin boys" alliance had branded him. His family was unable to escape the intergenerational trauma that cast a wide net over all their lives.

Our fourth session provided greater anchoring for S as he felt more of a somatic need for me and gave himself over to our relationship. Not a surrender, but rather a leaning into an organic need for self-preservation through mutual regulation. He began experiencing separation anxiety over the weekend breaks and soothed himself by remembering the comfort he felt with me Monday through Thursday. Becoming dependent upon me produced new and frightening feelings of unmet needs and loss. From time to time, he emailed me his thoughts and self-reflections during the weekend breaks. Knowing I would respond helped him bear his feelings as he found himself in my mind. S told me he couldn't fathom not having me in his life once the analysis ended.

And then his last dream of that week:

> *I am in my old house down in the basement where mother used to sit. I have a flashlight. Everywhere I turned the flashlight I see enormous spiders running along the walls. They were all over the place. I thought an army of harmless spiders. Then I woke up. The dream reminded me of one of my favorite children's books, BE NICE TO SPIDERS.*

He hadn't thought of the book in years and said, "Ah, the wisdom of children's books. Who gave it to me? One of the nannies? I must have been frightened all the time—this is why my hearing is so good." And then he tells me about counting my steps when he knows I am coming to get him.

Three days later he was dead of a ruptured aortic aneurysm.

Coda

S's seven-year analysis ended without warning, leaving me shocked and bereaved. He was a formidable man and a remarkable patient. I knew over time my memories of our work would fade, so I began writing this paper to mark our time together. As I wrestled with understanding the enormity of his neglect and abandonment, several theoretical perspectives were my guideposts. The analysis continued for me in writing this paper.

Surviving the enactment that almost blew up the analysis made us more resilient. For instance, although S never talked in detail about his relationship with his wife, he loved talking about her grandchildren from her first marriage, who recently moved back to the US with their parents after living abroad for some time and now visited often. Never wanting his own children, he was surprised how much he cared for the little ones. During their most recent visit, he colored in a coloring book for the very first time and told me how much pleasure he took in doing this with the youngest grandchild. I teared up, which S noticed and did not appreciate. "If you are trying to do 'empathy,' it's not working." Much to my embarrassment, I felt myself blushing and couldn't think for a moment. I felt shamed—he had put me in my place. I remained silent as I understood he experienced my empathy as pity, which was deeply shaming to him. A week after this, he bought a coloring book—his first one. He proudly showed me the pages that he had colored, all by himself. I said, "Good job, you colored within the lines!" He broke up laughing, and I knew all was well between us. I think we would have experienced many more of these kinds of enactments had he lived, bringing him more into the present with me. These moments of meeting would likely have become the wellspring of his healing.

Working with S was an unforgettable experience. I learned that my interpretations were for me, not for him. He was a natural hermeneut, and I adjusted by being in his space in a nonintrusive, curious way. I learned to be patient, opening my mind and heart to the unknown and staying in the flow of uncertainty. He didn't seek solutions or answers from me, only a safe place to lay his head. Throughout our seven-year journey, his rich dreams were the conduit to mining the depths of his psyche. The safety and resilience of our relationship facilitated the rebirth of his physical aliveness. As I was his witness to all of this, he found a different kind of partnership with me, a healthy twinship. This too was the wellspring of his healing.

Letting S go

There was so much mourning ahead of us—mourning the good mother and father he had been denied, the opportunities he couldn't reach, and the end of his analysis with me. I believe if we had had the good fortune to reach an agreed-upon termination, he would have experienced empathy for himself.

If S hadn't died, could he have relinquished his fetish for the long term? Could he have modified its use over time? I don't know. He said his chastity belt was "a second skin," part of his body, not some sex toy he could throw into an old box in his basement. But just when he seemed committed to change, he died. He lived his life too late.

Being in thrall to a disembodied object for over 35 years made it impossible for him to experience the sanctuary of being loved and truly loving another human being. Perhaps over time he would have found that. Our relationship gave him hope that change was possible—the past could become history. In those last six months without the chastity belt, he began to experience himself in the flow of time.

Notes

1 My office is in the backyard of my home, and I open the gate at the beginning of every session.
2 This is well captured in Bion's (1987) account of the "nameless dread" that lies in wait to be experienced and remembered in the transference to the analyst.
3 Stephen Seligman, personal communication 2024, suggested Titus Andronicus is the transformation of the cruel ruthlessness that was packed into and contained by the belt.

References

Bion, W. R. (1987). *Second Thoughts*. London: Karnac Books.
Celenza, S. (2014). *Erotic Revelations, Clinical Applications and Perverse Scenarios*. London and New York: Routledge.
Corrigan, E. & Gordon, P. -E. (1995). The mind as an object. In Corrigan & Gordon (eds.), *The Mind Object, Precocity and Pathology and Self-Sufficiency*. Northvale, NJ: Aronson.
Scarfone, D. (2015). *The Unpast: The Actual Unconscious*. New York: The Unconscious in Translation.
Seligman, S. (2016). Disorders of temporality and the subjective experience of time: Unresponsive objects and the vacuity of the future. *Psychoanalytic Dialogues*, 26(2): 119–128.
Williams, P. (2019). Isolation. *Psychoanalytic Dialogues*, 26(1): 1–12.
Winnicott, D. W. (1949). Mind and its relation to the psyche-soma. In *Through Paediatrics to Psychoanalysis* (pp. 243–254). New York: Basic Books, 1975.

Chapter 7

Delving into the never-ending challenge of reinventing psychoanalysis for severe perversion

Ofra Eshel

A theoretical-clinical context

My discussion of Margaret Rubin's "Calamities and Secrets, the Power of the Fetish" is based on her telling and moving paper and on my experience with cases of sexual perversion that I have treated over the years—severe cases that, to my mind, do not fall within the debate over whether they are a perversion or a "variance" (Stoller, 1974), or whether "perversion is us" (Dimen, 2001; Stein, 2003). Nor will I relate to patients whose perversity is expressed only in fantasy, in transference perversion, or in character perversion,[1] but to cases of actually acted, intense perversions of patients who have undergone years-long psychoanalytic treatments (analysis or intensive psychoanalytic psychotherapy). These patients actually belong to the type of perverts about whom Laplanche, de M'Uzan, and many other psychoanalysts write: "Doubtless, these patients—like most perverts—hardly ever consulted the psychoanalyst" (Laplanche, 1999, p. 201), and about whom Stoller adds, "Analysts dislike and fear perversion" (1991, pp. 53, 4). Yet, the patients addressed by Rubin and by me (Eshel, 2005, 2012, 2013a, 2013b, 2017a, 2019a) are perverts who did come, who stayed, and who underwent a long psychoanalytic treatment that delved into the heart of this difficult endeavor.

The psychoanalytic thinking of perversion has come a long way over the last 120 years, beginning with Freud's early writing (1905) on the subject. I will try to outline very briefly its theoretical landmarks and changes over the years, before moving on to the clinical discussion. The understanding of perversion in psychoanalytic thinking may be divided into two major frameworks: the drive model and the object-relations model, with a later addition of the selfobject model of Self psychology.

DOI: 10.4324/9781003674078-11

The first framework, historically, is **Freud's classical drive model** and its vicissitudes. Initially, Freud understood perversion from the economic point of view as a primary fixation of libido at pre-oedipal levels. Several years later (in the context of a growing interest in the ego), Freud came to recognize that perversions may serve as defensive formulations, especially against an Oedipus complex and castration anxiety, rather than simply as pieces of infantile sexuality that had evaded repression. In his later writings, especially in "Fetishism" (Freud, 1927) and in his important unfinished essay "Splitting of the ego in the process of defence" (Freud, 1938), Freud postulates other defenses in perversion: the "disavowal" of reality resulting in a "splitting" of the ego. These mechanisms bear significant resemblance to those found in psychoses. Yet, throughout his writing, Freud's theory of sexuality and perversion remains a drive theory, focusing on the Oedipus complex and castration anxiety.

Toward and during the second half of the twentieth century, a radically new way of understanding perversion evolved by way of **attachment and object-relations** theories. Rather than emphasizing endogenous drives, this perspective focuses on disturbed early mother-child relations, the mother's pathogenic role, and pathological ego or self-development. Here, perversion is regarded as a primary defense against intolerable, primitive, infantile anxieties and traumas and a self-induced survival solution to preserve a precarious, crumbling ego or self. This emphasis on primitive, psychotic anxieties rather than on neurotic Oedipal and castration anxieties brings perversion closer to psychoses. This "relocation" of perversion in early disturbed attachment or object relations greatly affected psychoanalytic thinking, especially in Britain, the U.S., and France.

Another important addition to the understanding of perversion took place with the development of American Self psychology, and its emphasis on the relation between the **self and its selfobject**—the primary psychological unit—in the child's early life. For Kohut (1972, 1977), most perversions are desperate attempts to repair the disintegrating self by means of perverse fantasies and activities. "The deepest analysis of … [perverse] manifestations does not, however, lead to a bedrock of drives, but to narcissistic injury and depression" (Kohut, 1977, p. 173). His followers, particularly Stolorow (1975a, 1975b; Stolorow et al., 1994) and Goldberg (1975, 1999), further explore the important narcissistic function of perversion, viewing it as an abortive, primitively sexualized attempt to restore and maintain the cohesiveness and stability of a precarious, crumbling self, or to defend against dreaded object situations and affects during the early pre-oedipal era.

Within the context of these main psychoanalytical perspectives on perversion and their clinical implications, Rubin's thinking belongs to the model of disturbed early-childhood relations. She focuses primarily on the patient's mother, whom I would describe, in Pontalis' words, as "the abyssal mother at the very bottom of depression"[2] (2003, p. 27). Pontalis uses metaphorically terms from marine Geography—"nautical depressions," taken from Baron (General Geography IX), in which depressions refer to the sunken parts of the earth's surface, situated below sea level and generally filled with water. There are three zones or levels of depth: a neritic zone (shelf zone) where all marine waters lie at the depth of less than 3000 meters; a pelagic zone (deep-sea zone) that extends from 3000 to 5000 meters; and an abyssal zone that includes large marine craters/abysses beyond 5000 meters deep, and this zone is the most dangerous and unknown.

Can analytic work reach these abyssal unknown and risky depths? Can something new come into being in those abyssal depths through the analytic work?

The radical change in the understanding of perversions is closely linked to the significant shift that has taken place within psychoanalytic thinking in general. As I described in Chapter 1, over the past decades, psychoanalytic thinking has moved theoretically and clinically into the traumatic depths of human experience and to emphasizing the traumatic of the real and the distortion of fundamental processes of relatedness. This shift has called for changes in psychoanalytic thinking and technique. Working psychoanalytically with non-neurotic patients and traumatic states of mind challenges traditional theory and practice. In my opinion, it forges an emerging dimension of analytic work of radical presence and transformative experiential human connection.

In this regard, my own way of working and thinking has delineated over the years a fundamental ontological-experiential dimension forged by the analyst/therapist's presence within the patient's experiential psychic reality and the grip of the analytic process, and the ensuing patient-analyst interconnectedness or "withnessing" that may deepen into at-one-ment with the patient's innermost emotional reality. The analyst gives himself over to becoming part of the patient's ongoing emotional reality and mental processes as an area of receiving, experiencing, processing, and transformation. This analyst-patient entity of experiencing and be(com)ing allows for traumatic experiences that the patient has been unable to bear to enter the now and be jointly met, experienced, and lived through t(w)ogether.

This way of working also resonates with the ontological shift currently taking place in psychoanalysis (Eshel, 2004a, 2017b, 2019a; Ogden, 2019), which reflects a deep commitment to the principle of *being and becoming in the experience* rather than epistemological (knowing) exploration and interpretation.

Fear of breakdown and the annihilated scream

At the beginning of her paper, Rubin conveys her

> hope to contribute to our understanding of the complex challenges of working with severely traumatized patients whose fetishism helps them bind the unbearable, keeping them locked in fixed and repetitive patterns of living in a world in which time doesn't pass.

Let me lay out some theoretical-clinical stepping stones toward this challenge of working with severely traumatized patients. Delving into the depths of early breakdown and madness, the unbearably painful last scream, and the immensity of the brokenness of a human psyche draws heavily, for me, on ideas from Winnicott's posthumous writings and Bion's late works, and also on Kinston and Cohen (1986) "primal repression," Williams (2022) "The authority of tenderness," and Grand (2000) "catastrophic loneliness." I will focus here specifically on Winnicott's groundbreaking late paper "Fear of breakdown" because, for me, this paper offers the closest understanding of severe perversion formation, as well as the way of working with it. Winnicott developed from the depths of his clinical experiences a radical new understanding of the meaning of early breakdown,[3] resulting from massive traumatic environmental-mother failure. His late (posthumously published) writings "Fear of breakdown" (1974/1963?), its continuation "The psychology of madness" (1965), and "The concept of clinical regression compared with that of defence organization" (1967), address the disastrous impact of being broken down at the beginning of one's life. The extreme primitive agony of early breakdown or madness is so unthinkable and "indescribably painful" that it cannot be experienced. Therefore, a new massive defense organization, displayed as the patient's illness syndrome, must be constructed against it in order to shut down and decimate this threat of unthinkable agony. With regard to severe perversions, I think that this massive defense organization is actually the *perversion*, which turns the patient from a passive victim of unbearable early damage, destruction, and helplessness into an active "doer," over and over again, while beneath it there yawns an abyss of devastation, inner death, and emptiness.

Consequently, the individual becomes imprisoned in an extremely dissociated, ever-present "unthinkable state of affairs that underlies the defence organization" (1974, p. 103), which has already happened, but since it has not yet been experienced, it cannot get into the past tense (*cf.* Scarfone, "the unpast," 2015), and is feared and compulsively sought after in the future. It is thus a timeless, ongoing catastrophe, then, now, about to happen—never and forever;[4] an endless impact on one's being that will continue until and unless it is relived and experienced.

According to Winnicott, there is a profound inner struggle in those depths of unthinkable agony of early breakdown or madness in treatment—a struggle between the buried, unexperienced dreadful past agony and a *basic urge* to experience it and thus "to be recovered in experience ... because it cannot be recovered in memory... [for] madness can only be remembered in the reliving of it" (1965, pp. 126, 125, italics in original). This evokes the fear of breakdown or of the return of the original madness, but also the patient's great need to reach to this original, unthinkable state of breakdown, to risk reliving and experiencing the early agony "for the first time in the present"—this time in treatment, with the analyst/therapist and his or her different holding and supplying "the auxiliary ego-supporting function of the mother" (1974, p. 105). Patient-with-analyst are given here a radical "new opportunity" to relive and experience t(w)ogether the feared, unexperienced, unthinkable, and unrepresented breakdown that is buried under the massive defense organization (here, the perversion). This goes further than Winnicott's fundamental model of therapeutic regression in the 1950s, where the hope is for a new opportunity for unfreezing the *freezing of the [maternal] failure situation*, re-experiencing it, and correcting the original failure situation. In fear of breakdown, the crucial question is could there be a radical hope—a "hope of getting at something here in the analysis that had never been before...Can something be created of nothing?" (Winnicott, 1986, p. 32).

Similarly, with regard to the screams of Rubin's patient, "the screams his mother never seemed to hear." Winnicott (1969, in an article written a year and four months before his death and also published posthumously) relates to "the scream that this patient is always not experiencing" because in childhood, their crying went unmet; "the child cried and the mother did not appear." For Winnicott, the scream that his patient "is looking for is *the last scream just before hope was abandoned.* Since then, screaming has been of no use because it fails in its purpose." The emergence of the patient's scream

> only becomes possible as a result of the analysis, in which hope about screaming returned... it is the only way to correct the failure of [the] last scream to work... Profound understanding on the part of the analyst on the basis of the material presented by this patient leads towards screaming, that is to say towards screaming again, this time with hope.
>
> (Winnicott, 1969, pp. 116–118, italics in original)

Late Bion in *Brazilian Lectures: 1973, Sao Paulo,* also relates to screaming:

> If I were a baby I could try screaming. If my mother was unable to understand that, I might become so frightened by the noise that I fell silent; then nobody, not even I, could hear my screams. I might have to find actions instead. If I grew up and found an analyst, I might try acting-out.
>
> (Bion, 1990, p. 48)

Let me now briefly return to the fundamental tenets I outlined in Chapter 1 concerning analytic work within severely traumatized psychic realities and the spectrum of analytic oneness. In recent years, inspired especially by Winnicott's (posthumously published) writings and Bion's radical late work along with my clinical experiences, I have further developed the dimension of patient-analyst interconnected being and experiencing, espousing deep-level patient-analyst interconnectedness or "withnessing" that may deepen into at-one-ment. I have emphasized the fundamental ontological experience of patient-analyst being-in-oneness at a primordial point of origin in order to be able to reach and transform the patient's most extremely dissociated, unknown, unrepresented states—mainly of nameless dread and mental catastrophe (Bion), unthinkable, unexperienced breakdown and madness (Winnicott), and "catastrophic loneliness" (Grand, 2000).

This work within difficult psychic realities pertains to the analytic work in the unrepressed unconscious.

The unrepressed unconscious

The unrepressed unconscious of non-neu*ro*tic patients and traumatic states of mind consists of psychic material that could not be repressed but is dissociated, split-off, and may become unrepresented. Thus, the unconscious in the realms of unbearable and catastrophic psychic trauma is no longer the repressed unconscious of psychoneurosis. It attempts to extend psychoanalytic practice beyond neurosis and beyond what were formerly thought to be the limits of analytic work. Taking this further (Eshel, 2023), it ranges from the *unrepressed realm, level I,* that is traumatically dissociated and unknown, to the deepest *unrepressed and unrepresented realm, level II,* of the most traumatic, unthinkable, and non-communicating emotional reality.

Analytic work in the unrepressed unconscious entails being in varying degrees of patient-and-analyst state of oneness and transformations in oneness, moving from patient-and-analyst *two-in-oneness (level I)* to *at-one-ment* with the patient's radically unknown, unrepressed, and unrepresented psychic reality (*level II*).

To sum up

The critical idea is that analytic oneness can open difficult-to-reach domains for further experiencing and transformation in treatment. Patient-with-analyst, or patient-at-one-with[5]-analyst, psyche-with-psyche, may undergo the devastating experience that made it impossible for the patient to be there and experience it alone. The unthinkable cannot be thought but only relived and gone through with the analyst. I believe that only by *being within* the patient's deep feeling states and their emotional impact can patient-with-analyst be given a new chance to relive and break through massive traumatic impacts.

The treatment

It is within this theoretical-clinical context that I will turn now to the intricate and difficult treatment of S with Rubin and follow the experience of her being there, growing deeply interconnected with the patient's emotional reality as the treatment unfolded, and the slow becoming of a lived emotional transformation.

S grew up with a mother who, from the very beginning of his life, was incapable of taking care of him; an unavailable mother, with whom the basic experience of "mother and child *live an experience together*" (Winnicott, 1945, p. 152, italics in original) could not take place. Her manic sexual and aggressive behaviors dominated his childhood. In addition, his father was either emotionally removed or given to violent rages, and S was traumatically overexposed to the oversaturating sexuality and bizarre behaviors of both his mother and father. He managed to survive his traumatic upbringing by withdrawing into a "universe of one"—the protected place for his isolated self, where the fetish he had constructed provided him some containment, safety, and control over the intense fear, neglect, and abandonment he felt but left him in a self state of hopelessness about anything ever changing. All these were sensitively handled and interpreted by his analyst, underscoring his distorted and constricted sexuality, aggression, and castration anxiety. But whenever she told him what she was thinking or offered an interpretation, his response was always, "I already knew that."

However, slowly, over time, with Rubin's continuous, sensitive emotional and caring involvement, another dimension was emerging in treatment, a dimension of concrete, non-epistemological, experiential, and emotional "contact with the thing itself." S, who sought analysis because his wife found him "emotionally unavailable" even after his first analysis and who offered facts about his family, education, career, and marriage with a complete lack of affect at the start of his treatment, seemed to slowly begin to change. Tears would come into his eyes. He would tear up when describing the ineffable beauty of the mountains surrounding the town where he grew up. Then he described a moving moment with a solitary horse that walked over to the fence where S was standing and gazing at him. "Spontaneously, he put his hand on the horse's head, feeling the heat and sweat of the horse. It was a moment of deep intimacy, and S began to weep. This was the first moment of palpable contact between us," writes Rubin.[6]

While early in his treatment, S had had a dream in which he was helping his analyst do an experiment on a person who seemed to be just a blank head with red and blue irises; now, step by step, he was confronting her with the essence of his catastrophe, with the enormity of his neglect and terror, and with his being lonely, lost, and empty. A little child was coming into being there-here, abandoned, lost, crying and screaming night after night, until his scream faded away and died out, and he had seized upon the fetish as a last bastion against this early breakdown and madness. Indeed, "the last scream just before hope was abandoned" (Winnicott, 1969, p. 117, italics in the original) now cried out from the depths of his metaphorical and concrete basement.

"Father, don't you see I'm burning?" whispered the burning dead child pleadingly, standing beside his sleeping father's bed and catching him by the arm, in the "moving dream" that Freud recounted (Freud, 1900, p. 509). But Rubin saw and heard S's pleading cry, and this opened up the possibility of facing the overwhelming nature and extent of the inaccessible, underlying past-but-ever-present catastrophe in his psychic reality. S was handing over to her, in a direct and concrete way, the relentless imprint of an early disaster on his ruined psyche and life: the true, actual meaning of devastation, desolation, and nothingness. Thus, it now became possible for the first time, in a "past-present actuality" (Eshel, 2004b), for Rubin to be with him within the realness of the breakdown and go through it, patient-*with*-analyst, "living the unthinkable, the unexperienced, and the unlived t(w)ogether" (Eshel, 2019b).

These are *crucial issues in the treatment of perversion*. Due to its dissociative, secretive nature, due to its being a self-induced survival solution of dissociative splitting and a compulsively driven and exciting ritual that does not truly change the deep inner stalemate, the pervert cannot be extricated from these repetitive cycles alone. But within and through the analyst's withnessing presence in the perversion-laden psychic space, as the patient slowly discloses his secrets, anxieties, feelings, and desires to the analyst, while also slowly and gradually revealing his concealed yearnings, a new inner voice is formed, heard, and evolves – though at times wallowing in dark, daunting, and dismaying burrows. *A present, alternative experiential-emotional reality is created*. It is a difficult treatment, most difficult. The psychic space of the treatment and the analyst's interconnected psyche are deluged with the effects of perversion, or with the search for a path in a world of despair, emptiness, and losing one's way, especially at the very time when the fierce perverse solution is destabilized and recedes.

Eigen writes similarly and poignantly: "More is involved than the capacity to know. …A capacity as deep or deeper than the sense of catastrophe must be called forth if healing or profound change is to occur" (1993, p. 219). "This kind of therapy involves commitment to deep experiencing… There is support deeper than anything one can hold onto" (2004, pp. 170–171)—"This collapse into being with another, the deepest states of the other" (Eigen, 2006, p. 38).

Indeed, this is *ontological-experiential* rather than epistemological-analytic work. The analyst's withnessing presence that may deepen into being *at-one*-with the patient's innermost emotional reality enables a new mobilization of the patient's primary and fundamental need for being and becoming with a holding, containing, and protective presence. At the same time, it also enables the *actual*[7] *becoming of a new, primary interconnectedness* with the analyst—who is "there to be used" (in the Winnicottian sense), steady, sustaining, and experience-near to the patient's needs, fears, and inability to relate.

This new possibility, which becomes part of the actual treatment reality, not only revives the original past situation but is also a process of becoming, a transformative process of change by breaching the limits of the patient's compulsive repetition and his catastrophic loneliness.

S's "universe of one"[8] is akin to the impenetrable "catastrophic loneliness" of the severely traumatized patients that Grand (2000) so hauntingly describes:

> The trauma survivor remains solitary in the moment of h[is] own extinction. No one knew h[im] in the moment when he died without dying; no one knows h[im] now, in h[is] lived memory of annihilation. This place where he cannot be known is one of catastrophic loneliness… Death has possessed h[im] in its impenetrable solitude.
>
> (p. 4)

Even when Rubin helped him sift through his messy stuff and they discarded the refuse together in her garbage bin, she felt that "his solitariness was heartbreaking." However, in the penultimate dream that S brought in the seventh year of treatment, this was profoundly changed, as Rubin, his analyst, *was there, within*. I quote this deeply stirring moment in full:

> [H]e had this dream: *"I was the sole survivor of a disastrous plane crash and was wandering around this huge debris field in high heels, littered in body parts and airplane parts. I am pretty sure I am a woman. You were the tv journalist interviewing me. I wondered if you knew I was a woman. I didn't remember the crash and didn't want to talk anymore. I was exhausted from screaming and wanted to go home but didn't know where that was. You said let's find you a place to sleep and rest."*

> As [Rubin] focused on the dream images, he said haltingly, "This is not a typical dream for me. I know I am having a lot of dreams of being a woman. But you wanting to take care of me deeply affected me. You heard my cries." His screams were finally heard. In his dream, S was able to begin to experience the catastrophe of his childhood that until now had been unthinkable. He had survived, but at such a cost.
>
> And he returned to these new feelings in a later session: "I think I am learning to reconnect to the suffering and pain I suffered alone. I think I am experiencing it now with you, and its different." He quietly cried—his silence enveloping both of us.

I would like to relate now to the issue of "addiction," which I regard very differently from Rubin. Rubin describes what happened with S regarding the fetish:

> "….All this lives within the configuration of the belt. *What can possibly replace my obsession?*" [he said]. Despite this, he tells me he would like to give up the belt. But is it possible? Being without it terrifies him. After some thought, I propose an addiction model might help him give it up for a time. How long, he wonders. I suggest we decide this once we see what feelings arise when he isn't using the belt, as it is the fetish that keeps him irretrievably stuck in the endless repetitions of his past. He nods anxiously but worries he won't know what to do with himself without his belts.

After this, Rubin recounts, S has a spate of dreams about being a woman as well as dreams and memories about his mad mother, and he seemed constantly annoyed with Rubin and was using the belt incessantly. Robin found his obsessive need to understand every nuance of the belt exhausting, but she wasn't sure what was going on between them. Had she sullied his relationship with the belt when she mentioned the word addiction? "You can't possibly understand me," S said furiously.

> When I was using the belt every day, you called it an addiction and said we should think of it that way. You had made an interdiction…. I've been angry with you for calling my belt an addiction, which I know it is. But what you don't understand is the belt is my way of surviving my parents' relationship.

But I feel that it is not about his "addiction" to the fetish that S is worried and hurt. He is afraid of becoming "addicted" to the treatment and to his analyst, that over the years of treatment became his new inner way of surviving his parents' relationship—years in which he slowly and gradually disclosed his painful memories, feelings of shame and dread, neglect, loneliness, desires, and concealed yearnings. These were all shared and revived in treatment, grasping and clinging to the analyst—to her attuned presence and the deep connection with her; one may say that his clinging to the analyst and the treatment replaces his clinging to the perverse solution. Thus, a possibility was created for experiencing and processing them and for the becoming of a different way of experiencing, being, and relating. All this enabled a profound change in the perverse essence, along with a slow, gradual entry of hope, life, and love—primary love (Balint, 1968) and primary relatedness (Kinston & Cohen, 1986), regression to dependence (Winnicott, 1954), and the vital neediness and vulnerability involved in this process. He was ready to give up the belt as a profound and daring act of trust and love for his analyst, but she did not understand. Rubin writes:

> Being in thrall to a disembodied object for over thirty-five years made it impossible for him to experience the sanctuary of being loved and truly loving another human being. Perhaps over time he would have found that, as our relationship gave him hope that change was possible.

But I feel that this nascent, primary love was already here, within.

S ran away from treatment for six weeks and came back; he came back to surrender—"the belt must go," he said—and gave himself over to their crucial relationship.

And Rubin describes:

> Our fourth session [that he requested] provides greater anchoring for S as he felt more of a somatic need for me and gave himself over to our relationship...He began experiencing separation anxiety over the weekend breaks... Becoming dependent upon me produced new and frightening feelings of unmet needs and loss... S told me he couldn't fathom not having me in his life once the analysis ended.

In the same vein, I understand his harsh reaction to Rubin's tearing up when he told her about his pleasure while coloring in a coloring book with his youngest grandchild and saying to her, "If you are trying to do 'empathy,' it's not working." I do not think that he experienced her response as pity. I feel that it was so touching and precious to him that he was very afraid of it being falsified and of being led astray.

"At the point of transition, when the analyst begins to get into contact with the patient's True Self, there must be a period of *extreme dependence*. Often this is missed in analytic practice... and the opportunity is missed" (Winnicott, 1960, p. 151, my italics). Later he powerfully adds, "Often at this point it is *a matter of life and death*" (1964, p. 98, my italics).

The death of the patient

"It is always dangerous to stir up the depths of the unconscious mind," writes Ogden (1989, p. 172). This is often the case when working with the patient's catastrophic near-death experience, at the edge of what can be spoken, felt, or even survived. Kinston and Cohen (1986) emphasize the dangers inherent in the abysmal depths of psychoanalytic work, postulating that whenever

> the traumatic face of primal repression is activated, death or near-death events like a major illness or serious accident to the patient become a real risk. These horrific events are characterized by being recognizably meaningful rather than merely coincidental. How avoidable such meaningful catastrophes are, is as yet unknown.
>
> (p. 339)

Eigen (2004) highlights another facet, which seems to me profoundly relevant here when working in the *liminal space between life and death*: "How much aliveness can one take?" he asks (p. 225).

At Bion's last New York seminar, New York—Five, in 1977, one of the participants poignantly described a psychotic man she worked with for many years. She almost gave up on this patient, and she suggested that maybe they could stop when he became better and started to have a normal life, but he said he could grow emotionally, and he indeed became better and better. He wanted to be able to love a woman and be married. When he was in his fifties, he fell in love. His therapist said that she could not believe it, but he married the woman, had a few very happy months, and then had a heart attack and died. He was only 56 when he died.

> Q[uestion]. Your question is, did you help him, or did you help him to death?
>
> O[bservation]. Yes. You can never know – which makes it rough.
>
> (1980, p. 71)

Eigen (2004), who was at this seminar, expands on this story in the epilogue of his book *Psychic Death*:

> Occasionally, a therapist experiences the miracle of such an individual growing more and more alive. In such cases not only is an individual helped to function better but also his or her emotional life evolves, becomes less stunted, more varied and intense. This is what Susan Deri experienced with her patient. He refused to give up on himself. She was loyal, devoted, and committed to him… but as he came alive, he wanted everything…. Then the unspeakable happened. He fell in love—and his love was reciprocated. I remember Ms. Deri describing her disbelief, her amazement: how could this happen? She credited her patient. It was he who kept going from level to level, wanting more, wanting whatever life could give. She was behind him, with him, each step of the way. But she never thought he had the capacity to support life at its fullest.
>
> There is no doubt that Ms. Deri felt his aliveness was too much for him. She felt guilty for—what?—not taking more care that he not become too alive? Surely, he had had decades of help to build up to it. How can one call his leap into life precipitous? Yet Ms. Deri felt the final burst of aliveness was too much for his physical being. His heart could not take its own opening.
>
> (2004, pp. 225–226)

Are we left with a deep and complex question regarding patients for whom the *change deadness-aliveness is radical*—can we or should we take more care that they would not get too alive, that they would not fall in love?

I join wholeheartedly with what Bion says at the end of this New York seminar; I feel that his words about pain, guilt, and bravery may also relate to Rubin's work:

> Bion: But somebody, sometime has to dare to investigate this terrible pain. What you are saying does involve the further investigation of the

guilt; not saying it does not exist or is not painful, but going on looking at it. It does involve standing up to the guilt of which one is aware. The same thing happens with other emotions; it is no good talking about brave man when he is avoiding being aware of the danger which he runs; he has to know it is a dangerous situation he is handling. What is known and felt to be dangerous and is still kept in view seems to me to be real bravery.

O. To be aware of the dangers of psycho-analysis and then to practice it –

B[ion]. And go on practicing it.

(1980, p. 74)

And go on practicing it—I cannot imagine better words to conclude this discussion. For the pain, the longing, the caring, the risk, the guilt, and the bravery are all in the meeting.

Notes

1 "perversion" throughout the paper refers to actual sexual perversion (cf. DSM IV-TR under Paraphilias) and not to the psychoanalytic expansion of the term over the last decades to perversion of the transference relationship and character perversion (especially in Kleinian thinking).
2 In marine geography referred by Pontslis, the abyssal zone denotes not only the deepest region of the sea but also its most dangerous and uninhabitable one. In this sense, Pontalis's "abyssal mother" might also be called 'abysmal'—her psychic depths both unfathomable and emotionally annihilating.
3 "Something surfaced from the depths of clinical involvement into conscious grasp and produced a new orientation to a whole area of clinical practice," wrote Clare Winnicott powerfully when the paper "Fear of breakdown" was published posthumously, in 1974.
4 In T.S. Eliot's (1942) words it is "Never and always": "Here, the intersection of the timeless moment … Never and always" (Little Gidding, p. 215).
5 "Be at one with" (Bion, 1967, 1970); "become 'at-one' with the patient's experience" (F. Bion, 1995, pp. 96, 107); "Being-at-one-with" (Winnicott, 1971, p. 94).
6 This brings to mind a similar story, "The horse" in Martin Buber's (1967) memoir *Meetings: Autobiographical Fragments*. Buber was raised by his grandparents because his parents separated when he was three years old and his mother left with her lover to Russia. He describes how, at the age of eleven, he experienced a moving moment of deep contact with a horse at the stable on his grandparents' estate.

7 *Actual* is intended here in its two meanings: "In the present and in the process of actualization, that is, trying to bring into existence what didn't happen" (Pontalis, 2003, p. 45).
8 I believe that of all mental disorders, the existential experience of the pervert is the loneliest, most isolated and alienated—both from the outside world and also within his/her internal world.

References

Balint, M. (1968). *The Basic Fault: Therapeutic Aspects of Regression*. London: Tavistock/Routledge.
Bion, F. (1995). The days of our years. In C. Mawson (ed.), *The Complete Works of W. R. Bion, Vol. XV* (pp. 91–111). London: Karnac, 2014.
Bion, W. R. (1965). *Transformations*. London: Maresfield Library/Karnac.
Bion, W. R. (1970). *Attention and Interpretation*. London: Tavistock.
Bion, W. R. (1980). *Bion in New York and Sao Paulo*. Perthshire: Clunie Press.
Bion, W. R. (1990). *Brazilian Lectures: 1973 Sao Paulo 1974 Rio de Janeiro/Sao Paulo*. London and New York: Karnac.
Buber, M. (1967). *Meetings: Autobiographical Fragments*. London and New York: Routledge.
Dimen, M. (2001). Perversion is us? Eight notes. *Psychoanalytic Dialogues*, 11: 825–860.
Eigen, M. (1993). *The Electrified Tightrope*. Ed. A. Phillips. Northwale, NJ & London: Jason Aronson.
Eigen, M. (2004). *The Sensitive Self*. Middletown, CT: Wesleyan University Press.
Eigen, M. (2006). The annihilated self. *Psychoanalytic Review*, 93: 25–38.
Eliot, T. S. (1942). Four quartets, little gidding. In *Collected Poems: 1909–1962* (pp. 214–223). London: Faber and Faber, 1974.
Eshel, O. (2004a). Let it be and become me: Notes on containing, identification, and the possibility of being. *Contemporary Psychoanalysis*, 40: 323–351.
Eshel, O. (2004b). From the "green woman" to "scheherazade": The becoming of a fundamentally new experience in psychoanalytic treatment. *Contemporary Psychoanal*ysis, 40: 527–556.
Eshel, O. (2005). Pentheus rather than Oedipus: On perversion, survival and analytic "presencing." *International Journal of Psychoanalysis*, 86: 1071–1097.
Eshel, O. (2012). A beam of "chimeric" darkness: Presence, interconnectedness and transformation in the psychoanalytic treatment of a patient convicted of sex offences. *Psychoanalytic Review*, 99: 149–178.
Eshel, O. (2013a). Patient-analyst "withness": On analytic "presencing", passion, and compassion in states of breakdown, despair, and deadness. *Psychoanalytic Quarterly*, 82: 925–963.
Eshel, O. (2013b). Tustin's "diabolon" and "metabolon" revisited: Further clinical explorations. *The Frances Tustin Memorial Prize, the 18th Annual Frances Tustin Memorial Lectureship in Los* Angeles, California, November.

Eshel, O. (2017a). Beyond sexuality, beyond perversion: The annihilated last scream. *Studies in Gender and Sexuality*, 18: 154–166.
Eshel, O. (2017b). From extension to revolutionary change in clinical psychoanalysis: The radical influence of Bion and Winnicott. *Psychoanalytic Quarterly*, 86(4): 753–794.
Eshel, O. (2019a). *The Emergence of Analytic Oneness: Into the Heart of Psychoanalysis.* London and New York: Routledge.
Eshel, O. (2019b). The vanished last scream: Winnicott and Bion. *Psychoanalytic Quarterly*, 88(1): 111–140.
Eshel, O. (2023). When deadness breaks in: Surviving, "Bemg-with" and a moment of "at-one-ment" in analytic work within deadness and emptiness. *Modern Psychoanalysis*, 47: 145–171.
Freud, S. (1900). The interpretation of dreams (Part 2). *SE*, 5.
Freud, S. (1905). Three essays on the theory of sexuality. *SE*, 7: 125–245.
Freud, S. (1927). Fetishism. *SE*, 21: 149–157.
Freud, S. (1938). Splitting of the ego in the process of defence. *SE*, 23: 273–278.
Goldberg, A. (1975). A fresh look at perverse behaviour. *International Journal of Psychoanalysis*, 56: 335–342.
Goldberg, A. (1999). *Being of Two Minds: The Vertical Split in Psychoanalysis and Psychotherapy.* Hillsdale, NJ & London: The Analytic Press.
Grand, S. (2000). *The Reproduction of Evil.* Hillsdale, NJ: Analytic Press.
Kinston, W. & Cohen, J. (1986). Primal repression: Clinical and theoretical aspects. *International Journal of Psychoanalysis*, 67: 337–353.
Kohut, H. (1972). Lecture 1 (January 7, 1972): Perversions. In P. Tolpin & M. Tolpin (eds.), *The Chicago Institute Lectures* (pp. 1–11). Hillsdale, NJ & London: The Analytic Press, 1996.
Kohut, H. (1977). *The Restoration of the Self.* New York: International Universities Press.
Laplanche, J. (1999). Masochism and the general theory of seduction. In *Essays on Otherness* (pp. 197–213). London & New York: Routledge.
Ogden, T. H. (1989). *The Primitive Edge of Experience.* Northvale, New Jersy and London: Jason Aronson.
Ogden, T. H. (2019). Ontological psychoanalysis or "what do you want to be when you grow up?" *Psychoanal Quarterly*, 88(4): 661–684.
Pontalis, J.-B. (2003). *Windows.* Trans. A. Quinney. Lincoln & London: University of Nebraska Press.
Scarfone, D. (2015). *The Unpast: The Actual Unconscious.* New York: The Unconscious in Translation.
Stein, R. (2003). Why perversion? Paper presented on the IARPP Online Colloquium, November 2003.
Stoller, R. J. (1974). Hostility and mystery in perversion. *International Journal of Psychoanalysis*, 55: 425–434.
Stoller, R. J. (1991). *Pain and Passion: A Psychoanalyst Explores the World of S & M.* New York & London: Plenum Press.

Stolorow, R., Atwood, G. & Branchaft, B. (1994). Masochism and its treatment. In R. Stolorow, G. Atwood & B. Brandchaft (eds.), *The Intersubjective Perspective* (pp. 121–126). Northvale, NJ & London: Jason Aronson.

Stolorow, R. D. (1975a). Addendum to a partial analysis of a perversion involving bugs: An illustration of the narcissistic function of perverse activity. *International Journal Psychoanalysis,* 56: 361–364.

Stolorow, R. D. (1975b). The narcissistic function of masochism (and sadism). *International Journal of Psychoanalysis*, 56: 441–448.

Williams, P. (2022). *The Authority of Tenderness*. London and New York: Routledge.

Winnicott, C. (1974). Editorial note. Fear of breakdown, D.W. Winnicott. *International Review of Psychoanalysis*, 1: 102.

Winnicott, D. W. (1945). Primitive emotional development. In: *Through Paediatrics to Psychoanalysis* (pp. 145–156). London: Karnac, 1992.

Winnicott, D.W. (1954). Metapsychological and clinical aspects of regression within the psycho-analytical set-up. In *Through Paediatrics to Psycho-Analysis* (pp. 278–294). London: Karnac, 1992.

Winnicott, D. W. (1960). Ego distortion in terms of true and false self. In *The Maturational Processes and the Facilitating Environment* (pp. 140–152). London: Hogarth, 1979.

Winnicott, D. W. (1964). The importance of the setting in meeting regression in psycho-analysis. In C. Winnicott, R. Shepherd, & M. Davis (eds.), *Psycho-Analytic Explorations* (pp. 96–102). London: Karnac Books, 1989.

Winnicott, D. W. (1965). The psychology of madness: A contribution from psychoanalysis. In C. Winnicott, R. Shepherd & M. Davis (eds.), *Psycho-Analytic Explorations* (pp. 119–129). London: Karnac Books, 1989.

Winnicott, D. W. (1967). The concept of clinical regression compared with that of defence organization. In C. Winnicott, R. Shepherd & M. Davis (eds.), *Psycho-Analytic Explorations* (pp. 193–199). London: Karnac Books, 1989.

Winnicott, D. W. (1969). Additional note on psycho-somatic disorder. In C. Winnicott, R. Shepherd & M. Davis (eds.), *Psycho-Analytic Explorations* (pp. 115–118). London: Karnac Books, 1989.

Winnicott, D. W. (1971). *Playing and Reality*. Harmondsworth: Penguin.

Winnicott, D. W. (1974). Fear of breakdown. *International Review of Psycho-Analysis*, 1: 103–107.

Winnicott, D. W. (1986). *Holding and Interpretation: Fragment of An Analysis*. London: Karnac Books and the Institute of Psycho-Analysis.

Chapter 8

Bearing the unbearable—in reply

Margaret Rubin

Dr. Eshel's paper offers an enriching and comprehensive view on the psychoanalytic treatment of perversions, dating back to early Freud through contemporary theories of treatment. Referencing Laplanche and Stoller, she observes that most perverts rarely seek analysis. Given that analytic work with perverse patients is the exception, I especially appreciate her position that psychoanalysis itself needs to change to effectively treat those suffering from severe trauma that underlies most perversions.

For myself, the Covid phenomenon loosened the boundaries of the analytic frame for the better. Seeing S in his home office via Zoom brought his interior states of mind into sharper focus, e.g., living in his mother's basement. Later, when he brought some of his "mementos" and "stuff" to my office to sort through and discard, he began the long process of organically feeling in possession of himself. I believe this was a precursor to giving up his accoutrement of restraints—eventually all the Slinkies that adorned his bookcases disappeared, and later the belts were put aside.

Dr. Eshel's (2019) ideas about "presencing" and "withnessing" influenced me throughout my treatment with S. Being quiet and patient with S, and myself, throughout this process was my North Star that permitted my presencing to lead to the analyst-patient interconnectedness or withnessing. Over time, this created the trajectory that allowed him to use me in the Winnicottian sense, as Eshel cogently describes. There is no 'how to do this' except to surrender to the uncertainty and unknown depths of despair in which the patient lives. As our "two-in-oneness" deepened, I knew we were moving toward a regression to dependency (Winnicott, 1954), and I worried about S's capacity to fully surrender to the process. What I hadn't fully realized was I had my own issues about surrendering and the responsibility it entailed. In one particularly quiet session, I feared I was failing

DOI: 10.4324/9781003674078-12

him. I stayed as steady as I could, listening and feeling into his feelings. When we approached the basic fault (Balint, 1992), I held my breath the way I did as a child when I dared to dive into deep dark water. I quote from Eshel's discussion: we relive together his "feared, unexperienced, unthinkable, and unrepresented breakdown that is buried under the massive defense organization (here, the perversion)." This nonlinear process continued until the end.

It was surprising to both S and me that his decision to stop using his chastity belts enabled him to quickly access his vitally alive self. He was ebullient as he began to experience present time without the past tugging him backward. He actually looked forward to tomorrow! Was I so caught up in his affective aliveness that I didn't respond to his concerns about the future when his analysis would end? Although he continued to tell me at different times that he dreaded this inevitability, I failed to hear his grief, as I always answered the same way—the analysis would end when he felt he had accomplished what he had hoped for, and the two of us would determine an end date. Writing this now, my response sounds glib. Eshel's suggestion that his addiction was to the analysis and to me is something I hadn't considered. I did know, however, that I and our relationship had become the conduit to his healing. What I didn't fully understand was that our two-in-oneness had moved him out of his solitariness in his universe of one and felt necessary to his going on being. Did this led to my off-handed response? Sporadic concerns about my responsibility in managing his regression to dependency felt overwhelming at times. Had he worried I was ready to move on, that our relationship was approaching its shelf life, and, once again, he'd be at risk of falling back into his echo chamber?

The day I learned of his death was our first session of the week, a Monday. S was always punctual, and if running even a few minutes late, he would text me saying he would see me in two or three minutes. Ten minutes after the hour I texted him saying, "I hope all is okay and you are on your way" (I thought to myself something I never think when a patient is late—I hope he's not dead). I didn't hear back from him. I told myself that perhaps he had an automobile accident, and I'd be hearing from him or his wife later. Late in the evening, I received a text from an unknown number, his wife's assistant, informing me he had died of a ruptured aortic aneurysm over the weekend, and I would be contacted later about a future memorial service. I was stunned, not only by the cold facts of the message, but that just like that he was gone. No good-byes. I was in disbelief that his life was over and our work together had come to such an abrupt and painful halt.

As I ruminate over Eshel's examination of the radical transition from deadness to aliveness, I wonder if his last few months of fervently believing in future possibilities had been too much for him. Had I known this without thinking it? Is this why the thought of his death popped into my mind? Was my enthusiasm for S too activating for his nervous system? Did this put him in a tailspin of dysregulation along with his fears of losing me? This remains unknowable.

Strangely, as I was finishing this response, the following lines of poetry by Swinburne were in my mind one morning upon awakening:

> For too much love of living, From hope and fear set free,
> We thank with brief thanksgiving whatever Gods may be
> That no life lives forever; That dead men rise up never;
> That even the weariest river winds somewhere safe to sea.

References

Balint, M. (1992). *The Basic Fault, Therapeutic Aspects of Regression*. Evanston, IL: Northwestern University Press with Brunner/Mazel.

Eshel, O. (2019). *The Emergence of Analytic Oneness, Into the Heart of Psychoanalysis*. London and New York: Routledge.

Winnicott, D. W. (1954). Metapsychological and clinical aspects of regression within the psycho-analytical set-up. In *Through Paediatrics to Psycho-Analysis* (pp. 278–294). Brunner/Mazel.

Afterthoughts

The generative power of living-through death in the work of Ofra Eshel

Dan Gilhooley

In the world of psychoanalysis, Ofra Eshel is the clinician's clinician. Having spent decades working with the most challenging patients, she is now recognized as a peerless practitioner. Working at extraordinary emotional depth—often across years of treatment described in detailed case reports—she shows how patients can transform and radically alter the course of their lives. How does she do it?

I

It begins by touching death.

Death is understandably unpopular. We prefer not to talk about it. Most of us structure our lives in ways that keep it out of sight, upholding the illusion that we'll live forever. And yet, we encounter death again and again over the course of our lives. In Israel, however, death is especially present. Many families carry direct memories of the Holocaust, and all live with the reality of recurring wars. Ofra has worked for decades within a culture marked by violent death—and she has developed a particular sensitivity to its psychic consequences.

So, how does death figure in Ofra's clinical practice? She draws on the late revolutionary work of her two inspiring figures in psychoanalysis, Donald Winnicott and Wilfred Bion (Eshel, 2017a). Within a Winnicottian model of deep shared regression, Ofra reaches back emotionally with her patient to a moment of traumatic breakdown—a personal catastrophe, usually occurring very early in life—when the patient psychically confronted extinction, an experience that left him or her lastingly crippled (Eshel, 2021).

Through this profound regression to the primordial origins of her patient's psyche, and drawing on Bion's conception of "transformation in O," Ofra enters a state of at-one-ment with her patient—she *becomes* the patient's psychic reality. As she writes, "at-one-ment with the patient's innermost experience is the only state of analytic being that can meet and transform core breakdown and mental catastrophe" (Eshel, 2019a, p. 2, 2019b). Referencing "chimeric" antibodies used in cancer treatments, Ofra sees her psychic presence slipping past the patient's defenses to form "an interconnected entity, *a new chimeric possibility*" (Eshel, 2019c, p. 93). It is through this deep analytic oneness that Ofra is able to deeply encounter the patient's traumatic experience of annihilation. Gripped by the pull of psychic death, she feels overwhelmed, helpless—yet present. Crucially, she *lives through* the patient's catastrophe not by dissociatingly surviving or defensively enduring it, but by entering into its full force while remaining emotionally present (Eshel, 2017b, 2023).

This *living-through*—rather than merely surviving—the annihilative experience becomes possible only through the depth of her psychic interconnectedness *with* the patient. And it is precisely *because* she is able to live through the catastrophe in this way that transformation becomes possible: through Ofra's radical interconnected presence, her patient too can undergo the experience of psychic death and re-emergence. As she writes, this shared regression "means experientially going through annihilation and death and coming forward again, but differently" (Eshel, 2017b, p. 37).

The patient rises from psychic death—like Lazarus. Death is transmuted into life. The transformation in oneness, born of this radical state of shared being, is sometimes so profound it borders on the miraculous. I believe that this rare capacity to work generatively within the realm of psychic death lies at the very heart of Ofra's clinical genius.

"Touching death" is the basis of human recovery and regeneration in archaic religions, a concept historian Mircea Eliade describes as the myth of eternal return. Eliade (1954) notes that human regeneration requires a return to a chaotic, formless state, a return to death and dissolution: "To recover vigor [human form] must be reabsorbed into the formless if only for an instant; it must be restored to the primordial unity from which it issued" (p. 88). Baptism is a symbolic form of *touching death* to initiate rebirth in Christianity, Judaism, Sikhism, and Hinduism. Eliade (1958) writes,

> Immersion in water symbolizes … a total regeneration, a new birth, for immersion means a dissolution of forms, a reintegration into the

> formlessness of [intrauterine] pre-existence; and emerging from the water is a repetition of the act of creation in which form was first expressed.
>
> (p. 188)

Ofra's conception of *living-through* death, developed from decades of clinical practice, is akin to these ancient religious models of regeneration following grievous injury and loss.

The idea of *living-through* death is elegantly simple, but it is also inherently dangerous. While *touching death* lies at the core of regenerative processes, in the somato-psychic realm, it also presents risks for both the patient and the analyst. Death is a powerful disintegrative force used to break down psychic structures in the creative process of growth and adaptation. It's a force of psychic dissolution akin to the biological process of apoptosis, programmed cell death, used in human growth and development. It's a mechanism essential to psychic change, but it's a dangerous tool to operate because its force can be overpowering. In this regard, consider Ofra's seven-year treatment of a young oncologist named Adam (Eshel, 1998, 2004, 2017b, 2019d, 2023). Ofra feels trapped and paralyzed by Adam's continuous descriptions of his passionate care for his dying patients, in which the life-and-death struggle has become absolute. She writes, "Nothing could compete with or break into this closed world of the struggle with death. I eventually became silenced, wordless" (2017b, p. 52). She continues,

> I found myself drawing back, pressing hard against the back of my chair as if trying to distance myself from him and his world of sickness and death, trying to … remove myself from the impact of this horror on my body and psyche.

Feeling utterly overwhelmed, Ofra says in distress, "The room today is full of cancer" (p. 53).

While being swept up in death, in this living through together within deep interconnectedness, Ofra experiences Adam's childhood immersion with an annihilating psychically "dead mother," a Holocaust survivor whose mind was consumed with sickness and death. Indeed, Adam's very choice of profession—to be trapped with death—was a perpetuation of his experience growing up in the "black hole of deadness" that was his mother's mind. But now, his profound emotional engagement with death within his analytic treatment becomes "a massive re-enactment of the traumatic past locked inside him" (p. 52). Within their interconnected experience of death, in an act of midwifery, Ofra's *living-through* death facilitates Adam's rebirth to a new psychic reality. Adam's emotional transformation was clearly felt. Noticing a change in her doctor, one of Adam's dying cancer patients declares, "You have learned to live" (p. 54). Within their be(co)ming-in-oneness, as Ofra becomes submerged in death, Adam arises alive.

Touching death can be gravely dangerous, bringing one to the very brink of life itself. In this volume (Chapter 6), when Margaret Rubin's long-term analytic patient begins to make notable progress, he dies suddenly of a ruptured aortic aneurysm. Could his death be related to the profound growth processes he was experiencing in his analysis? Quite possibly. The aorta is made up of three layers of tissue laminated together by connective tissue. Aortic aneurysms develop because of degenerative processes like atherosclerosis, connective tissue disorders, or irregular apoptosis (programmed cell death) leading to the loss of smooth muscle cells in the medial layer. Working within the somato-psychic realm, if these underlying disintegrative somatic conditions become amplified by a dissolutive psychic force introduced by *touching death*, this can overwhelm the body and contribute to an aneurysm rupturing. Psychoanalysis is a risky business. Therapeutically negotiating the disintegrative psychic force of death takes courage, skill, and strength of character. Ofra's work reminds us that this is a calling illuminated by hope but fraught with danger.

If you ask clinicians what they admire most about Ofra, they'll often speak of the profound emotional depth at which she is able to work and connect—the capacity to engage patients at their deepest levels. I take this to refer to the depth of regression she is able to reach with her patients. One reason her regressions run so deep is that Ofra plunges herself into the patient's subjective experience, sidestepping conceptions of her countertransference, which are inescapably subjective. She concurs with César and Sara Botella (2005), who write, "if the analyst's thinking can tolerate the movement of regression, without recourse to defensive *solutions* … culminating in a counter-transference meaning that turns the relationship into something 'already known,' he will find herself confronted by the formal regression of her thought, with the *unknown*" (p. 83, emphasis added). Eschewing the security of the 'already known,' Ofra pursues the great unknown, even the unknowable. Regressions to moments of annihilation likely propel the analyst back to the unknown prenatal origins of the mind—or to birth itself, the primal experience of life-and-death struggle. Similarly, confronting the profound reality of death may trigger a regression in the patient to that same original point.

What do we mean by "the origin of mind?" In terms of brain development, consciousness is possible during the seventh month of pregnancy, at which time the fetus is aware of its body, reacts to touch, smell, taste, and sounds, and displays social expressions in response to external stimuli (Padilla & Lagercrantz, 2020). Short-term memory, habituation, and learning all occur by the 30th week of gestation. And the development of these processes coincides with distinct sleep-wake cycles in the fetus, who begins to spend more and more time in REM-state sleep. During the final weeks of pregnancy, the fetus appears to be dreaming most of the time. So, with regard to the functioning of the brain, it's probable that the mind emerges in utero during the seventh month.

Both Bion and Winnicott considered undifferentiated early forms of mental experience or a prenatal state of mind. In *A Memoir of the Future,* Bion (1991) writes, "past experience with patients would have been less obscure if I had dared to imagine that the emotions displayed might be pre-natal" (p. 663). In *Experiences in Groups*, Bion (1961) "postulate[s] the existence of a proto-mental system in which physical and mental activity is undifferentiated" (p. 154). In groups, Bion believed unexpressed proto-mental phenomena become the basis of disease (Vermote, 2019). And Dolan Power (2025) suggests these proto-mental states are experienced by analysts working at the deepest levels with individual patients. Ofra cites Winnicott's advocacy for "'the experience of allowing a regression absolute full sway' (1954, p. 279), even to the earliest stages of prenatal life and birth" (Eshel, 2021, p. 172). So when we speak of depth in her work, I think we are referring to her remarkable ability to delve into and work within this state of "pre-existence"—reaching back to the very origins of mind, where an entirely different mode of experiencing and knowing comes into being.

Maybe Ofra's therapeutic shift from linguistically based interpretive reasoning to a form of *emotionally based knowing through being* in a state of at-one-ment actually reflects the holding mother's relationship to the emerging mind of the fetus. In the 1970s and 1980s, analysts wrote about "preoedipal" and "preverbal" transferences. I think Ofra leads us to consider a "prenatal" or "natal" transference state where at-onement is the essential, or the only, therapeutic stance.

In her essay "Being totally in the dark" (this volume, Chapter 1), Ofra claims regressing to the moment of her patient's profoundly traumatic experience,

> where the patient's emotional reality is mostly unthinkable, unexperienced, and unrepresented, necessitate—by definition—going beyond epistemological exploration to the analytic work of being and becoming with-in the patient's psychic reality, at-one-with the patient's innermost emotional reality. *The unthinkable cannot be thought, but only relived and gone through with or at-one-with the analyst.*
>
> (p. 17)

To my way of thinking, when coming into contact with death, the capacity to stay alive feels endangered by a pull toward dissolution and undifferentiated experience. Perhaps what Ofra describes as "unthinkable" or "unrepresented" is, in fact, the natural dissolution of thought that occurs when *touching death.* It seems probable that the same forms of undifferentiated thought characterize both the beginning and the ending of life. But proto-mental thought always possesses a natal sense of potential and produces an involuntary feeling of aliveness (Power, 2025). Regression similarly "carries with it, within the analytic process, *the hope and a new opportunity* for reliving and correcting the original maternal failure" (Eshel, 2021, p. 172). So regression to a proto-mental state is inherently hopeful, filled with possibility, creating new *beginnings,* and tilting toward life. It may seem paradoxical that *touching death* produces such generative potential, but that is the very nature of human regeneration, as Eliade (1954) reminds us. In *Death, Desire and Loss in Western Culture,* Jonathan Dollimore (1998) writes, "death is not simply the termination of life … but life's driving force, its *animating*, dynamic principle" (p. 192, emphasis added).

In his essay, "Into the wilderness with Ofra Eshel and her patient Clari" (this volume, Chapter 2), Charles Levin evocatively references Hannah Arendt's concept of *natality*—the innate human capacity to *begin anew.* In contrast to the absolute certainty of death, natality is "the miracle that saves the world, the realm of human affairs, from its normal, 'natural' ruin" (Arendt, 1958, p. 247). This innate human faculty is "an ever-present reminder that men, though they must die, are not born in order to die *but in order to begin*" (p. 246, emphasis added). Against the total predictability of death, natality represents the human capacity to act *unpredictably,* to introduce something unique—something *radically new* into the world—offering a new potential for freedom and innovation. Natality is the essence of human creativity, and Levin underscores that it is the fertile soil that Ofra and her patients tend.

II

Perhaps the most compelling and extreme evidence of the reality of at-onement comes from the telepathic dreams Ofra reports in her practice (Eshel, 2006). These dreams, reflecting a radical form of analytic oneness, testify to the profound interconnectedness she experiences with her patients. Her most fully described example, *"Where are you, my beloved?"* (this volume, Chapter 4), involves her work with Effie, a young mother who entered analysis feeling increasingly unreal and detached from her husband and daughter.

Effie's mother and grandmother, both Holocaust survivors, rebuilt their lives in Israel after losing their entire families. Effie's mother remarried and had two daughters, Effie being the youngest. But when Effie was ten months old, her mother's first husband—long presumed dead—suddenly reappeared, only to vanish forever. The shock plunged Effie's mother into a ten-month complete withdrawal that left a deep and lasting wound.

Decades later, in analysis, Effie dreamed of entering a cemetery at 4 o'clock, seeing her father's picture there, and feeling an unknown longing. Uncannily, this coincided with Ofra's own attendance at a memorial service for her father—at 4 o'clock the same day. How could Effie have known such intimate details of her analyst's life? Ofra writes, "It was as if she had entered my mind, had been in a place and time I had been in, inside the longing I had felt" (Chapter 4, p. X). It is breathtaking. We have no way of explaining how telepathic experiences occur. We only know that they happen. Each time they appear, they are mysterious, impossible, perhaps miraculous—certainly beyond scientific understanding.

Mary Tennes, the discussant of Ofra's telepathy article, remarks on the uncanny nature of such experiences: a feeling of anxious uncertainty about something real caused by an impossibility (Windsor, 2019). Tennes (2024) writes:

> Indeed, it is the breathtaking [impossible] interconnectedness implicit in the uncanny that can … make 'our hair stand on end,' a phrase also

> from Hamlet, spoken by the ghost, referring to the terror of that which lies beyond the ease of human comprehension.
>
> (p. 155)

Telepathic experiences reveal a frightening, unknowable reality that is both true and impossible.

Ofra considered Effie's traumatic beginning. At a decisive moment in her early life, Effie's mother was profoundly absent—what Ofra calls "absent-within-absence" because this absence was rooted in the mother's trauma: the devastating loss of her first husband. The catastrophic abandonment Effie endured so early may have sown the very ground for the telepathic experience that later unfolded. As Ofra writes, "Critical early catastrophe resides in a world of primal attachment, in a non-verbal or pre-verbal period, with an ensuing fixation on an archaic mode of communication"—*that is, telepathy* (Chapter 4, p. X).

Thus, when Effie sensed Ofra's emotional absence—perhaps preoccupied with her father's death—the telepathic dream burst forth. It functioned like a psychic search engine: locating Ofra, restoring their connection, and preventing the unbearable repetition of her original annihilating abandonment by the early mother. The telepathic dream reached and actualized a state of at-onement. "*The entire time I'm someone else,*" Effie said of her dream (p. X, italics in original). This statement—together with her uncanny sense of Ofra's longing at her father's grave—leaves little doubt about their becoming at-one. At-onement is real.

But why did this dream arrive on that particular night? Here, I think, we begin to "see double" (Botella & Botella, 2005). In the days preceding the dream, Effie described her husband finding her utterly detached, just as she sensed Ofra pulling away. Both women—like Effie's mother—were "absent-within-absence," reflections of one another. Why, then, did the dream take Ofra to her father's grave? Consistent with our motif of "touching death," Eshel observes that the five telepathic dreams she encountered in her practice were all "connected to matters of life and death in my world" (p. X). Effie's dream of standing at her father's tomb at 4 o'clock replays Ofra's own graveside experience—another doubling. The telepathic moment emerges as reproduction, a copy. It is as though Effie were saying, "At your time of traumatic loss I am here, at one with you. You are not alone." At this point, Effie becomes a mirror image of Ofra; their roles seem to reverse (Searles, 1979).

So why do we observe these numerous mirrorlike reflective forms in conjunction with the telepathic event? I believe they are a product of the deeply primitive early mind Ofra encounters and inhabits in states of at-onement with her patients. From the first moments of life, *imitation* is the infant's original and persistent mental act (Meltzoff, 2002; Meltzoff & Gopnick, 1993). Mind begins to form through the creation of mirrorlike reflections. Ofra keeps pushing us forward "into an enigmatic 'impossible' extreme of patient-analyst deep interconnectedness," to the very origins of psyche (Eshel, 2019e, p. 609).

III

Studying Ofra's work can itself be generative for clinicians. While writing this chapter, I gave my long-term supervision group a succession of her articles for possible discussion in our weekly sessions. I've worked with these analysts for 10–20 years, and they're each familiar with Ofra's work because I've regularly used her papers in my teaching. In this way, Ofra symbolically joined our group for the weeks I was writing this little essay, and she was welcomed as an old friend. One of the articles for possible discussion was her 2001 paper, "Whose sleep is it, anyway?"—The clinical material from that paper forms the basis for her current chapter, "Being totally in the dark," in this volume.

"Whose sleep is it, anyway?" describes Ofra's work with Clari, a patient suffering from recurring near-death dreams in which she feels over-powered by a suffocating force. Paralyzed, Clari struggles to keep breathing. These terrifying experiences made it impossible for Clari to fall asleep. Ofra was seeing Clari twice weekly in face-to-face psychotherapy when, during the fourth year of treatment, something remarkable occurred: for the middle 30 minutes of every session, Ofra fell into a deep sleep. This continued for several months, and she had no idea what was happening to her.

In my supervision group, as one of our sessions ended, members decided to discuss "Whose sleep is it, anyway?" during our next meeting. The group knew that our next session would coincide with a medical appointment that one of our members would attend earlier in the day with her husband, who was recovering from surgery and chemotherapy for pancreatic cancer. The purpose of this appointment was to review her husband's most recent scans, looking for a recurrence of his cancer. For the past year, in addition to discussing clinical matters in the group, she'd mourned the excruciating anticipated death of her husband of 40 years, sometimes surely *touching death.* At those moments, to the extent that we were able, we each went there with her. When our next meeting commenced, she was unexpectedly absent. Even more concerning, she was unresponsive to a phone call and text message we sent her. The group worried that some medical emergency had required her full attention.

With our anxiety about her husband's health looming in the background, the group turned to discuss Ofra's strikingly original paper—and the powerful, generative impact her sleeping had on her patient, Clari, whose therapy deepened in profoundly transformative ways as a result. The group felt buoyed. Our feeling of mortal dread lifted. We were inspired by Ofra's fearlessness, working in such a state of sustained uncertainty. Not understanding what was happening to her in each session, "in the grip of the unknown," Ofra persisted. Members were taken aback by the extraordinary vulnerability Ofra displayed. We wondered what cumulative effect such vulnerability had on Clari, session after session, week after week. In fact, Clari couldn't understand how Ofra dared to be "so very unprotected and exposed" (Chapter 1, p. 23). Clari could never dare to fall so soundly asleep. Was it Ofra's continuous profound vulnerability that liberated such changes in Clari? That's what seemed to be happening.

We were amazed by Ofra's deeply intuitive and creative work with Clari, which breathed life back into our group, "life after dread." Why were we so inspired? Was it her intuition or her creativity? I don't use the word "creative" lightly. My original training is in visual art, and I've spent the past 50 years as a practicing artist. It's from this perspective that I consider Ofra's sleeping through those sessions to be the most intuitively inspired psychoanalytic intervention I've ever encountered. I think Sandor Ferenczi would agree when I say Ofra Eshel is the Michelangelo of psychoanalysis. Ferenczi was the preeminent clinician among the first generation of analysts. Eshel has risen to that same stature today.

I read to the group a passage at the conclusion of her essay, "Being totally in the dark," where Ofra realizes that within her work with Clari an *act of faith* had emerged, born

> out of my fundamental, profound belief and trust in the psychoanalytic process, in the deep connectedness of patient-and-analyst, in myself as an analyst; and not less important—out of Clari's persistence in treatment which grew in great determination to intensify it, despite the dread.
>
> (Chapter 1, pp. 37)

Willing to work relentlessly, *totally in the dark*, Ofra intuitively gives herself over to a deep unconscious process. This is why my students and I study Ofra's work so intently. Sometimes, in her clinical examples, I feel like we are watching a miracle emerging before our eyes. Through her faith, Ofra becomes a "natural force," something larger than herself, actually "larger than life." It seems like life itself has enlarged her therapeutic capacity. Perhaps this "enlargement" is the basis of our feeling of inspiration. *In the grip of the unknown,* Ofra is willingly guided by an invisible unconscious force greater than herself in which she has deep faith. This is her source of clinical invention. I recognize this source as true, and I'm a true believer.

This is how one group of clinicians made use of Ofra's work. While touching death, in the face of dread, we were "lifted up," inspired by the infectious spark of life emanating from her creative work. As Ofra reminds us, as painful and frightening as it might be, it's only by traveling *in total darkness* to the boundary between life and death that we glimpse the true nature of reality. And only there do we get our chance to be reborn.

References

Arendt, H. (1958). *The Human Condition.* Chicago, IL: University of Chicago Press.

Bion, W. R. (1961). Group dynamics. *Experiences in Groups and Other Papers,* 6: 141–191. London, UK: Tavistock/Routledge.

Bion, W. R. (1991). *A Memoir of the Future.* London, UK: Karnac.

Botella, C. & Botella, S. (2005). *The Work of Psychic Figurability: Mental States without Representation.* London, UK: Routledge.

Dollimore, J. (1998). *Death, Desire and Loss in Western Culture.* New York, NY: Routledge.

Eliade, M. (1954). *The Myth of the Eternal Return: Cosmos and History.* Princeton, NJ: Princeton University Press.

Eliade, M. (1958). *Patterns of Comparative Religion.* Lincoln, NB: University of Nebraska Press.

Eshel, O. (1998). Black holes, deadness, and existing analytically. *International Journal of Psychoanalysis*, 79: 1115–1130.

Eshel, O. (2001). Whose sleep is it, anyway? *International Journal of Psychoanalysis,* 82: 545–562.

Eshel, O. (2004). Let it be and become me: Notes on containing, identification, and the possibility of being. *Contemporary Psychoanalysis,* 40: 323–351.

Eshel, O. (2017a). From extension to revolutionary change in clinical psychoanalysis: The radical influence of Bion and Winnicott. *The Psychoanalytic Quarterly,* 86: 753–794.

Eshel, O. (2017b). Into the depths of a "black hole" and deadness. In A. Reiner (Ed.), *Of Things Invisible to Mortal Sight: Celebrating the Work of James Grotstein* (pp. 19–41). London, UK: Karnac.

Eshel, O. (2019a). *The Emergence of Analytic Oneness: Into the Heart of Psychoanalysis*. London, UK: Routledge.

Eshel, O. (2019b). Two-in-oneness: Transformations in O. In *The Emergence of Analytic Oneness: Into the Heart of Psychoanalysis* (pp. 27–43). London, UK: Routledge.

Eshel, O. (2019c). A beam of chimeric darkness: Presence, interconnectedness, and transformation in the psychoanalytic treatment of a patient convicted of sex offenses. In *The Emergence of Analytic Oneness: Into the Heart of Psychoanalysis* (pp. 92–116). London, UK: Routledge.

Eshel, O. (2019d). Into the depths of a "black hole" and deadness. In *The Emergence of Analytic Oneness: Into the Heart of Psychoanalysis* (pp. 44–65). London, UK: Routledge.

Eshel, O. (2019e). Would clinical psychoanalysis shy away from delving further into the unknown? On the mystery of telepathic dreams. *International Journal of Psychoanalysis*, 100(3): 608–610.

Eshel, O. (2021). Winnicott's clinical theory of regression: A radical new opportunity through the fundamentals. *Journal of the American Psychoanalytic Association,* 69: 167–179.

Eshel, O. (2023). When deadness breaks in: Surviving, "being-with" and a moment of "at-one-ment" in analytic work within deadness and emptiness. *Modern Psychoanalysis*, 47: 145–171.

Meltzoff, A. (2002). Elements of a developmental theory of imitation. In A. Meltzoff & W. Prinz (eds.), *The Imitative Mind* (pp. 19–41). Cambridge, UK: Cambridge University Press.

Meltzoff, A. & Gopnick, A. (1993). The role of imitation in understanding persons and developing a theory of mind. In S. Baron-Cohen, H. Tager-Flusberg & D. Cohen (eds.), *Understanding Other Minds* (pp. 335–366). Oxford, UK: Oxford University Press.

Padilla, N. & Lagercrantz, H. (2020). Making of the mind. *Acta Paediatrica: Nurturing the Child,* 109(5): 883–892. https://doi.org/10.1111/apa.15167.

Power, D. (2025). The breath of life: Bion's concept of the proto-mental. In D. Power & D. Power (eds), *The somato-psychic realm: Analytic receptivity and resonance* (pp. 1–18). London, UK: Routledge.

Searles, H. (1979). Concerning therapeutic symbiosis: The patient as symbiotic therapist, the phase of ambivalent symbiosis, and the role of jealousy in the fragmented ego. In *Countertransference and Related Subjects* (pp. 172–191). New York, NY: International Universities Press.

Tennes, M. (2024). “Tell all the truth but tell it slant:” Psychoanalysis and the uncanny. *Contemporary Psychoanalysis*, 60: 146–166.

Vermote, R. (2019). The protomental matrix. In *Reading Bion* (pp. 56–57). London, UK: Routledge.

Windsor, M. (2019). What is the uncanny? *British Journal of Aesthetics*, 59(1): 51–65.

Winnicott, D. W. (1954). Metapsychological and clinical aspects of regression within the psycho-analytical set-up. *Collected Works,* 41952–1955: 201–217. L. Caldwell and H. Robinson (eds.) (2016). Oxford, UK: Oxford University Press.

Index

Note: Page numbers followed by 'n' refer to notes.

For Product Safety Concerns and Information please contact our
EU representative GPSR@taylorandfrancis.com Taylor & Francis
Verlag GmbH, Kaufingerstraße 24, 80331 München, Germany